Chemical Dependency
A Family Affair *Leova.*

D1644027

Olivia Curtis

Brooks/Cole Publishing Company

I(T)P® *An International Thomson Publishing Company*

Pacific Grove • Albany • Belmont • Bonn • Boston • Cincinnati • Detroit • Johannesburg • London
Madrid • Melbourne • Mexico City • New York • Paris • Singapore • Tokyo • Toronto • Washington

Sponsoring Editor: *Eileen Murphy*
Marketing Team: *Michael Campbell,*
  Christine Davis
Editorial Assistant: *Susan C. Carlson*
Production Editor: *Keith Faivre*
Manuscript Editor: *Linda Purrington*

Permissions Editor: *Connie Dowcett*
Interior Design: *Christine Garrigan*
Cover Design: *Vernon Boes*
Art Editor: *Jennifer Mackres*
Typesetting: *Joan Mueller Cochrane*
Printing and Binding: *Webcom*

Credts continue on page 134.

For more information, contact:

BROOKS/COLE PUBLISHING COMPANY
511 Forest Lodge Road
Pacific Grove, CA 93950
USA

International Thomson Editores
Seneca 53
Col. Polanco
11560 México, D.F., México

International Thomson Publishing Europe
Berkshire House 168–173
High Holborn
London WC1V 7AA
England

International Thomson Publishing GmbH
Königswinterer Strasse 418
53227 Bonn
Germany

Thomas Nelson Australia
102 Dodds Street
South Melbourne, 3205
Victoria, Australia

International Thomson Publishing Asia
60 Albert Street
#15-01 Albert Complex
Singapore 189969

Nelson Canada
1120 Birchmount Road
Scarborough, Ontario
Canada M1K 5G4

International Thomson Publishing Japan
Hirakawacho Kyowa Building, 3F
2-2-1 Hirakawacho
Chiyoda-ku, Tokyo 102
Japan

Printed in Canada.

10   9   8

Library of Congress Cataloging-in-Publication Data

Curtis, Olivia.
    Chemical dependency : a family affair / Olivia Curtis.
        p.   cm.
    Includes bibliographical references and index.
    ISBN 0-534-35583-8
    1. Substance abuse—Treatment.   2. Substance abuse—Patients—
—Family relationships.   3. Family psychotherapy.   I. Title.
RC564.C87   1998   98-21058
616.86'0651–dc21   CIP

About the Author

Olivia Curtis received her master of science degree in interdisciplinary counseling from Eastern Washington University, Cheney, Washington, and a liberal arts degree from Evergreen State College, Olympia, Washington. She has worked in the chemical dependency field since 1981, initially as a counselor working with alcoholic/addicted people and later as treatment director. In that capacity she provided clinical supervision to chemical dependency counselors, independently worked with family members, and conducted family interventions. She also had a private practice specializing in family-of-origin, parent–child counseling, and advanced recovery issues. Between 1986 and 1996, she taught chemical dependency and the family and counseling courses part-time at local community colleges. In 1988 Curtis assumed the position of executive director of a nonprofit chemical dependency treatment facility. She currently performs the same function as associate director, in the facility enlarged by a merger with another nonprofit agency in 1996.

Contents

Chapter Four

The Family as a System   33

Chapter Five

Elements of the Emotional System   43

Chapter Six

Family Organizational
Structure and Development   54

Chapter Seven

Chemical Dependency's
Disruption of Organization   66

Chapter Eight
Critical Issues in Chemically Dependent Families   75

Chapter Nine
Family Assessment   91

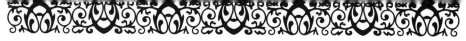

Preface

For a period of ten years I was engaged by a local community college as a part-time instructor of courses for students aspiring to be chemical dependency counselors. In teaching the "Chemical Dependency in the Family" course, I could never find just one text that covered the material I felt was important to convey to my students. To provide an adequate basic understanding of family system dynamics and how chemical dependence affected those dynamics, I had to use two or three texts.

This endeavor was prompted by my interest in developing one text that was more comprehensive for that course. This text is not intended to provide instruction specifically on how to counsel families. It is, however, intended to summarize, fairly comprehensively, the development of family theories, the structure of a family system, how chemical dependency affects a family, and how such addiction is woven into the family system. Although initially intended as a text for aspiring chemical dependency counselors, it is equally suitable as a supplemental text for other social science courses. The book also should interest members of the general population seeking to understand the subject.

I am grateful to the following reviewers of the manuscript for their helpful comments and suggestions: Sandy Croswaite, Pierce College; Harold Doweiko; Iris Heckman, Washburn University; Ron Jackson, University of Washington; Dorothy Neufeld; Eileen O'Mara, University of Nevada–Reno; Willie Whitfield, Ivy Tech State College.

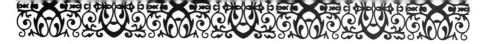

Chapter One

The Development of Family Therapy

Seeing family therapy as a specific discipline is a fairly recent development. For generations, cultural and religious premises, generally inflexible in nature, governed family rules and parenting methods. Traditionally, families did not "hang out their dirty laundry," and the consistently misbehaving child was often considered a "bad seed." The extended family or the church usually dealt with emergent problems within the family or with an individual family member.

As extended families became less accessible for advice and problem resolution, many parents sought assistance elsewhere. As various psychological and developmental theories were introduced, professionals became more aware of situations that might not previously have been considered problems for which people might seek help. However, the significance of family dynamics as a contributing factor in behavioral and emotional development was not fully recognized until about the mid-1950s.

Several factors have influenced the need for family therapy. Societal standards and expectations—always changing, and sometimes rapidly—can inflict considerable stress on families. Societal norms frequently conflict with a family's established values. And living standards and family ideals have changed significantly over the past half century.

Horne and Ohlsen (1982) have noted many social changes that have contributed to family issues. A greater sense of sexual freedom is now afforded by birth control pills and devices. Women's working outside the home has become generally accepted. Escalating costs of living, along with a search for instant gratification for some, has often required both parents to work. There has been a tremendous increase in single-parent, stepparent, and interracial families, all of which may be vulnerable to added stress.

There has been a shift in the family roles of parents: Women work more outside the home, and fathers have become willing to be more involved in a nurturing parental role. Greater mobility and technological advances have drawn many people away from rural environments to more urban, industrialized ones. Being geographically removed from their extended families, members such as grandparents or aunts are not available to help with raising children. Many of these changes have contributed to shifts in family structure.

Societal change and external forces, real or perceived, can place a tremendous demand on the family to constantly change and adapt to its members' needs. Support and education for mothers—who were the primary caretakers for children—in child-rearing and health care were once provided by the extended family and neighbors. Today, community mental health centers, support groups, churches, and pediatricians have largely taken over these functions. For some families, the number of extracurricular activities within the school system requires increased parental involvement. Or, conversely, children may have very little parental involvement and supervision. Peer influence relating to adolescent drug abuse and gang involvement can also place additional stress on families.

Mass media have influenced society's values, beliefs about right and wrong, attitudes about how families should be, and what constitutes the American dream. In the past, especially before World War II, the family locus of control was more often on the father, who dominated and assumed responsibility for family decision making and earnings. He generally dictated policy and had the buying power. The locus of control is now often divided and shared by both parents or held by a single custodial parent.

Aside from all the external forces with which families must learn to cope, there are all the normal developmental crises that families confront. Establishing a new family, children being born, children leaving home, changing a career, and facing retirement are all events that any family may confront. Families often no longer have extended family to help them manage stress, grief, child-rearing, and financial insecurity. Young adults, facing busy schedules of work, family taxi service, and parenting, often seek outside help in dealing with family issues.

Americans are now living longer and experiencing longer periods of retirement. Adult children often face the dilemma of how to deal with aging parents. Older parents may face escalating costs of living in retirement, and may feel confusion and anger about being set aside by their busy adult children. Many families have not been able to adapt rapidly enough to cope effectively with all the pressures created by both the external factors and developmental issues that they confront.

HISTORICAL REVIEW OF
FAMILY THERAPY DEVELOPMENT

Although it wasn't until the 1950s that family therapy began to fully emerge, the concept of working with or considering the family as a group evolved from the numerous small-group studies that began during the 1920s. Researchers conducted studies of natural groups in society in the hope that by gaining an understanding of group interaction they could learn how to solve social problems. Some of the group discussions held with patients led to the development of group psychotherapy. Among the more prominent of these small-group researchers was Kurt Lewin (1951).

Lewin's studies looked at the organic interactions between individuals and their environment. Among other findings, he concluded that a group, as far as dynamics are concerned, is a coherent whole and is more than merely a collection of individuals. Lewin and his colleagues observed that the actions of one member impacted or influenced all the other members. In other words, the causal relationship was circular, rather than a direct, separate interaction between one individual and another. He also found that group discussions were more effective than individual instruction in getting people to change ideas and social behavior. Lewin's group of researchers concluded that to accept and initiate change, group members must have their established beliefs and behaviors challenged.

In 1946, Lewin (1951) and his colleagues developed T-groups. Although T-groups were designed initially as a way to learn about group behavior, their focus shifted to helping participants clarify and realize their own goals. The T-group eventually evolved into the encounter group, which had the purpose of encouraging personal growth and enrichment. Conclusions drawn from Lewin's studies suggested that the principles of group interaction could be applied to conjoint family therapy.

Wilfred Bion (1984), another influential researcher of group dynamics, also made some basic assumptions that could easily be applied to family therapy. According to him, most groups become diverted from their primary goals by engaging in one of three specific patterns. First, group members may become involved in conflict. When confronting or avoiding the conflict, rather than problem solving, becomes the primary focus of the group participants, Bion describes the group as a *fight–flight* group. A second diversion, a *dependency* group, involves a dependent relationship of the members on the leader. In a *pairing* group, members are more interested in the social context for the group.

A number of other students of group dynamics have focused on such concepts as group cohesiveness, the relationship of leadership and power, and authoritarian versus democratic groups.

According to Nichols (1984), Alfred Adler organized the first child guidance clinics with the intent of providing an atmosphere of optimism and confidence for the participants. He founded his ideas on the belief that because emotional disorders usually began in childhood, the best way to prevent mental illness was to treat the problems of children. Initially working in Vienna, Adler introduced the child guidance movement into the United States in the 1920s. Aside from the parents providing a description of the problem behavior, the therapist usually saw the symptomatic child apart from the parents. The focus of treatment in the child guidance clinics was the child's symptomatic behavior. Therapists used various techniques to help alleviate the child's feeling of isolation and inferiority. The goal of treatment was to alter the child's behavior and create a personal internal locus of control. The belief underlying this practice was that this treatment would result in the child ultimately working out a healthy lifestyle.

Initially, the Adlerian therapists tended to consider the parents responsible for the child's problems. A social worker usually saw the mother separately. The purpose was primarily to reduce emotional pressure, redirect hostility away from the child, and to modify parenting attitudes. This model considered the family to be an extension of the child, rather than the other way around. Eventually the therapist saw the parents with the child, but only as an adjunct to one-to-one therapy with the child.

Child guidance workers gradually came to the conclusion that the real problem was not necessarily the child's behavior or symptoms. Rather, tension within the family needed to be addressed. Emphasis shifted to helping patients better relate to their families. According to Nichols (1984), Nathan Ackerman initially fostered the practice of treating the whole family.

Concurrent with the many small-group studies and the child guidance movement, studies were being conducted on families that had a schizophrenic member. Gregory Bateson and his colleagues looked at patterns of communication that might explain the origin and nature of schizophrenia in the context of the family system (Bateson, Jackson, & Weakland, 1963). They hypothesized that the family achieves stability by a feedback loop that monitors the behavior of the family and its members. In other words, family member interactions work in a circuitous or reciprocal fashion. These researchers theorized that whenever the family is threatened or disturbed, something must occur to move the family toward achieving **homeostasis,** or balance. A common tactic might be a child's disruptive behavior intended to interrupt the parents' fighting. Such disruption would tend to unite the parents, if only in concern for the child. The child's symptomatic or disruptive behavior thus functions to preserve the family's equilibrium.

The Bateson group also concluded that psychotic behavior could result from a child having to cope with confusing communication within the family, or with a double bind (Bateson, Jackson, Haley, & Weakland, 1956). Children can be caught in a double-bind situation when they pose questions to their parents that the parents consider threatening or contradictory and therefore impose injunctions on the children.

For example, a child, frequently hearing his mother complain about his father's drinking and behavior, may ask her "Why is Father so mean when he drinks?" Mother promptly replies authoritativly, "How dare you talk about your father that way? He's sick. You'd better show more respect for your father, or you'll be punished!" In this instance, the child learned that although his mother was unhappy about the drinking, it was not okay to see what she was seeing. Somehow his father's mean behavior commanded respect, and he had no right to question a parent's behavior.

A scenario I witnessed some years ago is another example of a double bind. A 2-year-old was repeatedly climbing up on the coffee table and jumping off. His mother each time told him, "You don't climb on the table," and threatened to spank him, although she never did. At some point his uncle sat down in a chair near the table, and the mother, laughing, told the child, "Jump on Uncle Steve." The conflicting message the child received was that somehow it was wrong to climb on the table but it really didn't matter because the threatened consequence was never carried out. At any rate, it was appropriate and funny to climb on the table when he could jump on Uncle Steve.

Such situations give children double messages, and so the children learn to look for a hidden meaning in what is being communicated by others. They grow up unskilled in the ability to communicate, to determine what people really mean, and in the ability to relate effectively with others. Nichols (1984) describes this double-bind phenomenon as having six characteristics:

1. Two or more people are involved in an important relationship.
2. The relationship is a repeated experience.
3. A primary negative command is given, such as "Do not do X, or I will punish you,"or "If you don't do X, I will punish you."
4. A second command is given that conflicts with the first, but at a more abstract level, and is also enforced by punishment or perceived threat. This second command is often nonverbal, and frequently involves one parent negating the command of the other.
5. A third negative command exists that prohibits escape and also demands a response.
6. Finally, once the child is conditioned to perceive the world in terms of a double bind, the necessity for every one of these conditions to be present disappears, and almost any part is enough to precipitate panic or rage.

Murray Bowen (1978), while working with schizophrenics at the Menninger clinic in Topeka, Kansas, began to conceptualize schizophrenia as having to do with an unresolved symbiosis between mother and child. Bowen became increasingly aware of the disparity between what he was observing with family dynamics and the then prevalent focus of psychoanalysis on the individual. From these studies, he began to appreciate families as "systems." Conclusions from his studies formed the basis of his family systems theory, to be further discussed later.

In 1956, members of Bateson's group began to see parents along with their schizophrenic child. Jay Haley, one member of that group, also considered the issue of struggles for power and control among people (Haley, 1976). A number of other individuals also were involved in studying schizophrenic families during this time frame, among them Theodore Lidz, Lyman Wynne, and R. D. Laing (Nichols, 1984).

Nichols speculates that John Elderkin Bell, Don Jackson, Nathan Ackerman, and Murray Bowen share the credit as originators of family therapy. Other significant pioneers of family treatment were Jay Haley, Virginia Satir, Carl Whitaker, Lyman Wynne, Ivan Boszarmenyi-Nagy, James From, Gerald Zuk, Christian Midelfort, and Salvador Minuchin.

Family therapy provided a whole new approach to understanding human behavior. Previously, therapists had considered that behavior was purely a product of individual personalities as influenced by discrete past events. Family therapy recognized, in addition, that dominant forces of personality development evolve from interactions within the family system. The principle of family therapy assumes that any attempt to understand people must be set in the context of their families.

THE TREATMENT OF THE CHEMICALLY DEPENDENT

Prior to the establishment of discrete alcoholism treatment, alcoholics were often placed in mental institutions, without much evidence of success. The prevailing belief was that alcoholism was a moral issue and that the alcoholic was weak in character. Quite often, by the time this placement was considered necessary, the alcoholism was generally so far advanced that, in all likelihood, not very many had an intact family.

For many years alcoholism and drug addiction were usually treated separately. As more research data became available, alcoholism treatment facilities began to incorporate treatment for addiction to "other drugs." Although addiction to each specific drug presents some discrete factors to be addressed during treatment, there are more commonalities among the addictions than differences. "Alcoholism treatment" emerged into "alcoholism and other drug addiction treatment." Currently it is more commonly referred to as "chemical dependency treatment." Generally, the terms "addiction" and "chemical dependency" are considered to be synonymous and to include alcoholism.

Many chemical dependency treatment professionals had previously considered it inappropriate, during early recovery, to deal with issues of the chemically dependent's family of origin. They generally believed doing so would diminish the individual's focus on personal responsibility for recovery and would drastically interfere with that person's recovery. However, many chemically dependent patients appear "stuck" in their emotional development and must face some of those issues in early recovery. Some people are unable to achieve stable recovery until they address critical and traumatic family-of-origin issues that seem to block recovery.

The focus of treatment, of course, was the affected individual and the cessation of drinking. Family or family developmental issues were not a consideration. Eventually therapists recognized that many treated alcoholics were not always having the desired success in recovery. This failure was largely caused by the numerous adjustment or readjustment problems that arose within their families after treatment. Moreover, family members were simply unable to adjust to the change in family dynamics from that previously associated with the drinking behavior. Family members were often left to face major issues such as their own unresolved anger and guilt and no longer having the drinking to blame for family problems that likely still existed. Residual fear and uncertainty also remained about whether the alcoholic could remain sober.

Today, the concept is emerging that healing for the chemically dependent person needs to occur in a multidisciplinary framework. Although most family-of-origin work should be delayed for later recovery, issues related to possible recovery failure should be dealt with early on. Treatment for the chemically dependent person must focus on the addiction as the primary problem, but should also be integrated with individual developmental psychology and family systems theory.

According to McNeece and DiNitto (1994), through the 1960s treatment for the nonalcoholic spouse continued to consist of a separate program concurrent with that of the alcoholic. This procedure was being followed despite the facts that the systems and behavioral theories already looked at the interactive, reciprocal nature of family processes and that conjoint therapy had already developed. Most family therapists lacked education on alcoholism and, when they noted an alcohol problem, they referred clients to alcoholism treatment programs. Also, alcoholism counselors seemed to avoid the family perspective, often because they lacked adequate training in that area or believed that perspective was incompatible with the disease model of alcoholism in which they were trained. Family members had little or no opportunity to become aware of how their own interaction patterns might have contributed to the family's dysfunction.

Gradually treatment professionals began to examine the significance of the interplay among other family members that not only contributed to but perpetuated family dysfunction, whether or not the dependent was actively using. Counselors often made referrals to Al-Anon for the spouse, but many spouses refused to get involved. Family members generally seemed unable to grasp that the family's problem entailed more than the drinking. Families subscribed to the general myth that once the drinking stopped, the family problems would disappear. It was difficult for family members to comprehend that they also needed to change old patterns to live happily and productively, with or without the alcoholic. Eventually many treatment facilities made provisions to treat other family members—at least the spouse. However, the treatment generally afforded the rest of the family was only ancillary to the alcoholic's treatment process.

FAMILY TREATMENT IN CONJUNCTION WITH ALCOHOLISM

Rivers (1994) provides a review of the history of alcoholism family treatment as presented by Steinglass in 1977. The initial concept of dealing with alcoholism and the family, beginning in the 1930s, considered family issues as likely being responsible for the alcoholic's drinking. Therapists emphasized specific family patterns that appeared to contribute to alcoholism, and geared treatment toward helping the alcoholic recover.

Until the development of family therapy in the mid-1950s, alcohol counselors generally conducted alcoholism treatment. Any treatment of the family focused primarily on the family behaviors that appeared to sustain the alcoholic's drinking. In the meantime, professionals in the family therapy field focused more on the communication and interaction patterns of the entire family as they interfaced with family problems.

According to this review, later in the development of family treatment focus was placed specifically on the manner in which wives initiated and maintained their husbands' drinking. Most clinicians held the position that women married alcoholic males to meet their own psychological needs. The focus was still being placed on the alcoholic marriage and the influence of wives in being responsible for and maintaining their husbands' drinking. Somewhat conversely, sociologists held the view that the wives were reluctant to give up their role as the better functioning partner. Because they couldn't trust their husbands' new-found sobriety, they often sabotaged the husband's recovery to avoid giving up these roles.

Whalen (1953) proposed that there are four types of wives of alcoholics. She suggested that a husband's continued drinking was maintained by the neurotic needs of his wife. Her study, however, preceded the women's movement and was based on a limited sample from her own clinical experience. She did not take into consideration that some wives of alcoholics might demonstrate no pathology. She also did not consider there might be more categories or various progressive stages. Nor did the study recognize that the alcohol abuse itself may lead to drastic shifts in the relationship between the marital partners. Unfortunately, her assertion that these types were typical for marriages in which alcoholism was present became widely accepted at the time. This labeling probably further stigmatized the alcoholic and the alcoholic family.

Whalen not only characterized her assumptions about these four types of wives, but also assigned somewhat descriptive labels to them. According to her, *Suffering Susan* has low self-esteem and self-worth. Mistreatment by an alcoholic husband helps to confirm her self-image as an unworthy person and to ensure that she remains miserable. *Controlling Catherine*, because she wants to control the marriage relationship, marries an inept, unassertive male. She is openly critical of her husband, but maintaining his drinking increases her control as her husband's alcoholism progresses. *Wavering Winnifred*, out of her own dependency needs, will choose a weak, inadequate husband. In doing so, she can feel secure in the relationship so long as his drinking continues and she can feel that he cannot get along without her. *Punishing Polly*, being both envious of and resentful toward males, will risk marriage only to a man who is inadequate and vulnerable and then constantly belittles him so his only recourse is to rebel by drinking.

Jackson (1954) reached somewhat different conclusions from her three-year study of wives who attended weekly Al-Anon meetings. Instead of deep-seated neurotic needs leading to alcoholic marriages, she found wives were sharing a similar set of adjustment stages in reaction to their husbands' drinking. She suggests that instead of different types of wives, as identified by Whalen, there were different stages in the wives' adjustment to the alcoholic marriage. Rivers (1994) has summarized those stages:

Stage 1: Tension and embarrassment are created by the drunken episodes at the beginning of the husband's abusive drinking. By both of the partners denying the problem exists, they avoid facing the problem.

Stage 2: As the drinking increases, the family becomes more socially isolated. The wife attempts to keep others from knowing by covering up the husband's drinking. The family becomes more centered around the drinking, leading to increased intensity and conflict in their interactions. The wife develops self-pity, and the husband becomes more resentful at her attempts to control his drinking.

Stage 3: As it becomes disorganized and experiences increased problems with the children, the family gives up. Sexual activity between the marital partners is limited, and violence frequently occurs. The wife becomes more resentful and begins to question her sanity. Family members feel helpless. Outside help may be sought, but this may result in the wife feeling guilty because she is unable to handle the problems herself.

Stage 4: As the husband appears to require more caretaking, the wife assumes responsibility for the family. She gains more confidence in her abilities as she successfully meets each new challenge. The children experience fewer problems, and the family stabilizes.

Stage 5: With some initial difficulty and considerable self-doubt and conflict, the wife and children leave the alcoholic husband.

Stage 6: The mother and children establish themselves without the alcoholic.

Stage 7: If he can demonstrate that he can remain sober, the alcoholic husband may be allowed to return. Reasserting himself in an adult role, however, is difficult.

Jackson's conclusion also seems somewhat limited. It does not consider that different families may follow different courses in the progression of alcoholism. It also does not take into account that the entire family may get help before the progression reaches a family breakup.

Rivers (1994) relates that Steinglass reported that the next step in developing family treatment for alcoholism was providing concurrent therapy for alcoholics and their wives, although in separate therapy groups. Ewing, Long, and Wenzil (1961) at the University of North Carolina Medical School studied 32 married alcoholics and 16 of their wives. Their purpose was to compare treatment outcomes between alcoholics whose wives were involved and those whose wives were not. In this regard, all participants received the same treatment format and were followed on a long-term basis. The Ewing group's study revealed that (p. 215, quoting Rivers) "alcoholics whose wives were in treatment (1) stayed in treatment longer, (2) had significantly improved control of drinking, and (3) had major improvement in 'marital harmony,'" compared to those whose wives did not participate. Other researchers obtained similar results.

Family therapy and substance abuse treatment was kept separate for several years. Until the 1960s and 1970s many family therapists, psychologists, social workers, and psychiatric training programs ignored substance abuse, generally considering it a nuisance. Alcohol-based family treatment had focused more on adapting existing individual and group therapy techniques to improve treatment outcomes for the alcoholics. Concurrently, professionals working with schizophrenia, psychosomatic disorders, and dysfunctions of adolescents were developing techniques to improve a variety of family-based problems.

According to Rivers (1994), among the first to suggest that alcoholism was a family disorder, and that therapy should focus on changing family members' interactions, were Ewing and Fox, in 1968. They contended that the alcohol abuse maintained the family emotional homeostasis. They concluded that if only the alcoholic changed, the spouse might resist the change. Therefore, it was necessary to work with both husband and wife to help them "learn to interact with each other without the presence of alcohol" (Rivers, 1994, p. 215).

According to Rivers (1994, p. 216), further findings of Steinglass, Davis, and Berenson in 1975 supported the theory that "the alcoholic's drinking might be highly adaptive for the family." Some families typically experienced depression, fighting, and emotional distancing among members. However, when alcohol was present they were often observed, instead, to be warm and caring. Steinglass looked at alcohol use in terms of how it affects family interaction and how it is integrated into family life. He considered that alcohol "might assume such a central position in the lives of some families as to become an organizing principle for interaction life within those families" (1977, p. 279).

Steinglass suggested that treating the family as a unit focuses on modifying and changing the interaction among family members to improve their flexibility and functioning, rather than on only the alcoholic. The therapist must first determine how the drinking behavior fills an adaptive role for the individual and the family, and must identify the maladaptive outcomes of drinking. Then the alcoholic can be helped to learn appropriate alternative behaviors to replace the drinking.

Rivers notes that the next step in working with alcoholic families was to provide conjoint family therapy involving two or more members of the nuclear family and/or the extended family. Steinglass's review of a clinical report by Meeks and Kelly (1970), although involving only five alcoholic couples, showed that conjoint family therapy seemed viable. Applying Satir's (1967) family therapy model in an aftercare program, they addressed issues such as clarifying interaction conflicts, improving and opening up communication, and developing an understanding of how intrapsychic issues affected interpersonal conflicts.

Steinglass expanded on this approach by involving multiple couples and multiple families at the same time, working with ten middle-class intact couples who, despite the fact that one member was alcoholic, had stable economic and family lives. In each couple, the alcoholic had failed previous attempts at treatment. This particular program did not require abstinence and used the intoxicated behavior of the alcoholic as an adjunct to treatment. Treatment involved both partners and focused on the "interactions between alcohol use, intoxicated behavior, and how the couple related to each other." On completing the program, all ten couples reported having experienced improved family functioning.

Currently there is widespread recognition that family treatment should at least be an integral component of treatment for the chemically dependent. It would be even more preferable, of course, to have greater availability of programs providing family treatment beyond that fundamental involvement. Some treatment programs and facilities are devoted specifically to families with a chemically dependent member. Unfortunately, there aren't enough to meet the actual need. This scarcity is particularly apparent for families with limited financial resources.

There is yet another obstacle to families receiving treatment. Public information about chemical dependency's negative influence on families has been more readily available in recent years. Nevertheless, despite this increased public awareness that alcoholism/addiction is a disease, many family members are reluctant to become involved in treatment, even when the chemically dependent is receiving treatment. This reluctance is often caused by the stigma of alcoholism/addiction being perceived as a moral issue, or because they feel the need to control their own environment and handle matters on their own, despite their apparent lack of past success. There is also still a prevailing belief among some family members that once the drinking stops, all family problems will be resolved. However, an encouraging trend, most likely resulting from the Adult Children of Alcoholics movement, is that more individuals are seeking help for themselves so that many dysfunctional patterns will not be carried into another generation.

Chapter Two

Theoretical Approaches to Family Treatment

Family therapy provided a whole new approach to understanding human behavior. Previously, behavior was considered to be a product of individual personalities as they were influenced by discrete past events. Family therapy recognizes instead that the dominant forces in personality development lie within interactions in the family system. Therefore, attempts to understand people must be made within the context of their families.

A number of theoretical approaches are directed toward using family therapy in alcoholism treatment. Rivers (1994) summarizes those of Dulfano and Kaufman, as follows.

DULFANO'S APPROACH TO FAMILY ALCOHOLISM

Dulfano's (1985) approach comes from a perspective that views the family as a system. He contends that the separate and differing expectations brought into a marriage must be resolved so that both partners preserve their individual identities. As children enter the unit, the couple faces learning new tasks and new patterns of relating to one another. The feedback loop within the unit makes any change in the role of one member also change other members. Such change in interaction patterns can then evoke additional change in the originating member. Throughout its development, the family constantly needs to change and compromise, while simultaneously maintaining stability for the individual members.

Dulfano notes that the family is a social group in which people learn to love, care for others, and get their own needs met. The functioning of this primary social system affects the manner in which individuals grow and develop. Alcohol abuse can drastically affect this system by distorting family relationships. For example, the parents may organize their interactions around the alcoholic's behavior. Any changes in the parental subsystem can affect the children. If one or both parents decline in functioning, the children may be forced to assume adult roles, which deprives them of nurturing and of having their needs adequately met. An older child who finds satisfaction in an assumed parental role may encourage younger children to remain more immature. Such role distortions produce an atmosphere in which children cannot trust and learn to form appropriate close relationships with other people. The children can be severely affected under these conditions. They may continue these patterns in their adult lives and reenact them in their own nuclear families.

Dulfano contends that the cessation of drinking can threaten other members of the family as much as it does the alcoholic. If the alcoholic successfully changes his or her behavior, the family system may respond by interacting in patterns that encourage a return of the alcoholic behavior. To remove the family's pressure on the alcoholic to continue drinking, Dulfano believes the system must change structurally.

Although Dulfano designs each intervention with an alcoholic family individually, his therapeutic approach focuses on the cessation of drinking, and on holding the alcoholic responsible for doing so. Alcoholism is thus removed from its central place in the family. He targets for change those family transactional patterns that trap family members in roles that hamper growth. Simultaneously, he encourages individual growth of family members that is not based on dysfunction created by alcoholism.

Dulfano initially assesses the position of each family member, to determine how alcoholism has distorted family relationships. Therapy focuses on how family members are interacting with each other at the present time. Therapists work on interactional patterns of the marital relationship and the couple's parental roles with the children. The children are helped to let go of inappropriate assumed roles, and to become more involved in age-related activities and roles and less involved in the parents' problems.

KAUFMAN'S APPROACH TO FAMILY ALCOHOLISM

Kaufman (1985) combined aspects of structural systems and behavioral and psychodynamic approaches in his approach to working with alcoholic families. He suggests that there are four different types of alcoholic families and provides intervention strategies for each.

The Functional Family System

In the functional family, the alcoholic member drinks because of neurotic problems or circumstances external to the family. The family members, in most respects, live a happy, stable life with good relationships among them, and have minimum visible conflict. This type of drinking problem is not likely to be presented for treatment.

For this type of family, Kaufman suggests family education so that the members "may get involved in 'educative-cognitive exploration' of the roles each member plays in the family." They may also become more aware of observable family interaction, which in turn leads to exploring implicit family rules and the family's expectations of behavior. As a result, the family can develop family contracts and practice new behavior roles.

The Neurotic, Enmeshed Family System

For the "neurotic, enmeshed" family, drinking behavior has disrupted normal family functioning, resulting in conflict and role shifts as family members adopt new responses to the behavior. Sexual dysfunction and alcohol-related debilitating illnesses may affect the alcoholic member, further stress the marriage, and force more role changes for family members. Communication is ineffective, and members project conflict onto other family members.

In such a family, members feel guilty and responsible for the alcoholic and his or her drinking, and for each other. Each marital partner tries to gain control over the other. The drinking partner attempts to gain control by drinking and by becoming passive-dependent. The nondrinking partner attempts to control the drinking, perhaps by being blunt, by dominating, or by becoming a martyr. As the drinking progresses, the family makes major role changes. The nondrinking spouse may take over responsibilities of the other or may encourage an older child to take over. The alcoholic becomes more isolated and resentful. The children may suffer abuse. The father's abuse is likely to be verbal, with the possibility of physical or sexual abuse. An alcoholic mother is more likely to neglect.

Intervention for this type of family may include education and cognitive reeducation, but may also involve explicit family psychotherapy. Treatment may need to include extended families. Therapists encourage family members to become involved with people and groups outside the nuclear family, such as an extended family member, new friends, and community groups. Involvement in Alcoholic Anonymous and Al-Anon can help family members work toward emotional detachment from the nuclear family.

The Disintegrated Family System

The disintegrated family shows more advanced **enmeshment.** Kaufman suggests that the functional alcoholic family can also deteriorate into this stage. Although the family has so far had a reasonable family life, it has now broken down completely and the alcoholic is likely to be temporarily out of the home.

Treatment for this group usually begins with the alcoholic, although the therapist explores potential ties to family and friends. Once sobriety and social stability have been established for a period, but still before family reuniting is considered, therapy involving the nuclear and extended family can occur. Family roles and relationships need to be redefined and modified whether or not the alcoholic is reunited with the family.

The Absent Family System

In the absent family scenario, the alcoholic's drinking has resulted in a complete separation from the family. Any relationships the alcoholic now has are likely to be alcohol related. Although reconciliation with spouse and children is unlikely for this group, contact with the family of origin may be reestablished at some point.

Treatment of this group must be directed toward developing new social networks and social systems. Although some alcoholics who have been permanently separated from their families may eventually learn to interact in new social systems and establish new functional families, many will be unable to do so.

THERAPEUTIC MODELS OF FAMILY TREATMENT

The preceding theoretical scenarios, although differing in some respects, provide fairly clear pictures of alcoholic families. Rivers (1994) also examines different models of family treatment. Current family therapies have developed from somewhat different theoretical perspectives, which determine specific treatment philosophies for alcoholic families. McCrady (1989) divides them into the following three categories and comments on the research on outcomes for each.

The Disease Model

The disease model looks at alcoholism as a family disease. Nonaddicted family members are defined as *codependent*, which implies the tendency to possess many of the same traits observed in the alcoholic. Some treatment programs deal with the development of dysfunctional family roles, faulty communication, and changing family patterns in relation to the alcoholic. However, nonalcoholic family members are usually treated separately from the alcoholic. Treatment generally involves education about alcoholism and how it affects families. Referrals are made to groups such as Al-Anon or Adult Children of Alcoholics for ongoing support. Although likely to be of a shorter duration than for the alcoholic, some programs offer inpatient treatment for family members.

Although the disease perspective is widely employed in the United States, relatively little research conducted has been aimed at outcome. McCrady contends that the existing studies are limited and have lacked control or comparison groups. Most research has relied on self-report measures and does not provide information on the impact of treatment on the whole family. It also fails to link treatment with the drinking behavior or adjustment of the alcoholic.

The Behavioral Model

The behavioral perspective considers that abusive drinking behavior is maintained by a number of reinforcement contingencies, both from within and outside the family. The focus here is on how one member's behavior triggers the behavior of the partner, and on how the partner's response reinforces the first member's behavior. For example, the alcohol may allow the drinker to be less inhibited or more assertive, which reinforces the alcoholic. Simultaneously, the nondrinking spouse may decrease negative responses toward the drinker. The primary task of this model is to "develop ways to replace positive reinforcements gained when drinking with reinforcers that occur in response to sober behaviors." Treatment also focuses on the nondrinking partner's ineffective coping responses. It may include individual behavioral treatment with the alcoholic concurrently with the marital therapy. It looks at the locus of complaint and focuses primarily on isolated bits of specific behaviors or specific events within the context of the family. The therapist identifies targeted behavior and determines specific objectives for reducing or eliminating the identified behavior.

According to McCrady, although this model is used less frequently to treat alcoholism and the family, it has been the basis of the best research studies. This model has had favorable results in treating couples and appears to have the greatest impact in helping alcoholic couples deal with the threat of relapse after treatment. McCrady suggests that this model has gained little acceptance in the past in alcohol treatment programs because of the limited training of alcoholism counselors.

The Family Systems Model

The family systems perspective emphasizes family organization and the need for homeostasis. It holds that interaction patterns, family structure, and family roles are all organized around the abuse of alcohol.

In treatment, specific concerns or issues of the family members are set aside to focus on the interactions of the family unit. The drinking problem, how drinking changes the family's interaction patterns, and what family members' contribute to the drinking problem are dealt with in the family unit. Treatment goals include redefining family roles, modifying alliances between family members, and changing communication patterns. It looks at the family as an interacting system from a multigenerational or historical perspective. Of major concern are the impact that alcoholism has on children and the factors that contribute to the transmission of alcohol problems from one generation to another.

Many alcohol therapists have enthusiastically adopted the family systems perspective. According to McCrady, however, there has been relatively little research to substantiate its effectiveness. It has been speculated, however, that this approach with couples leads to a better treatment outcome than individually oriented treatment.

THE FAMILY AND DRUGS
OTHER THAN ALCOHOL

The research conducted for drugs other than alcohol, particularly in relation to the family, is not as abundant as for alcohol alone. A private treatment facility would likely see a different type of clientele from that of a nonprofit organization providing publicly funded treatment. Considering my own clinical observations, not research, I've not seen much difference in the impact of other drug abuse on family dynamics, from what has previously been described for alcoholism. Strictly in personal observation of individuals presenting for treatment, however, some questions perhaps warrant consideration with regard to families and drugs other than alcohol:

1. Do family members, particularly parents, increase their attempts to protect a drug-using family member, because of the illegality of these drugs, because they are unwilling to do anything to risk having their loved one incarcerated?
2. Do some family members consider the abuse of other drugs to be much more serious than the use of alcohol, and are they therefore more inclined to become concerned about the user sooner?
3. Is there a higher incidence of drug use (than of alcohol use) by both partners in a relationship, using the same drugs?
4. Are drug users who have completely disengaged from their families, possibly because of the illegality of the drugs, more numerous and also younger than alcoholics?
5. Does the higher cost of illegal drugs create a more rapid and greater financial hardship?

6. Particularly among the financially disadvantaged, are there more instances of drug-using parents who have lost custody of their children due to the parents' drug use, than among alcoholics?

It may be necessary to consider these factors in addressing not only the needs of the family but also, perhaps, where the emphasis of treatment is initially placed. For instance, if a family is experiencing a great deal of shame related to the addiction stigma, encouraging them to let the dependent experience the consequences through incarceration— yet another stigma—will likely only compound their shame and guilt. Therefore, it may be prudent to set that particular emphasis aside until the family has achieved more stability in other areas.

Aside from these factors, the denial related not only to the dependent's use but also to the contribution of all members to the family dysfunction seems to prevail as with alcoholism. In other words, family secrets, minimization of the problem, enabling behavior, blaming, and self-blame also exist.

Chapter Three

Family Therapeutic Theories

Specific therapeutic models or styles used in working with families vary depending on the therapist's own philosophical belief, personality, and effectiveness. Provided here is merely a brief descriptive outline of a few major theories of family therapy. These therapeutic models are only representative of all those available to the practitioner. Each has its own distinctive techniques and philosophy with regard to working with families. However, all the theoretical approaches discussed here share the belief that family interactions determine how the individual members and the family as a unit will function.

EXPERIENTIAL/SYMBOLIC THERAPY

Experiential/symbolic therapy evolved over a number of years from a variety of Carl Whitaker's professional experiences. Its name derives from the perspective that people's experience occurs apart from their consciousness and that their experience can be accessed symbolically, through nonverbal play (Keith & Whitaker, 1982). Play in this context is characterized by family members taking on "as if" positions in switching roles with other members. This provides an experience of knowing how one is perceived by another.

View of the Family
The experiential/symbolic approach categorizes families on a continuum of being healthy to dysfunctional, and self-actualizing to growth inhibited. This theory considers that family rules and regulations, rather than being specifically stated, have their origin in the covert and implied operation of the family and are largely expressed in a manner of living. This approach holds that the healthy family has a "sense of an integrated whole" that functions as the control system to uphold the family's unity and to promote change.

By contrast, the unhealthy family has a very limited sense of unity. Rules and roles are inflexible. Dysfunction in a family is related to the struggle over whose family of origin the new family is going to model itself after. This struggle results in a family growth impasse. Often the only person in the family who believes in the "spirit of the family" is either the one creating the greatest distraction and on whom the blame may be placed, or the one held in esteem by the family. The actions of the scapegoated one stress the family. The actions of the other help the family cover up anxiety and unhealthiness. Expression of individual differences, to renegotiate role structure and role expectations, and the freedom afforded healthy family members, are not possible in the unhealthy family.

Major Tenets
A major presumption of Keith and Whitaker is that "it is experience, not education that changes families." Health is a process of perpetual becoming, and dysfunctional families become growth inhibited. They believe that the therapeutic process must involve an attempt to identify the meanings behind behaviors as they are symbolically played out.

Goal of Treatment
The goal of treatment is to increase the creativity of the family and its members and to get the family members to believe in themselves as a unit while simultaneously gaining freedom to develop as healthy individuals.

Therapeutic Style
The experiential/symbolic model generally uses cotherapists. The preference is to work with the extended family along with the nuclear family as a unit. Although considering the historical significance of specific issues, therapists tend to separate the generations. Therapists function as coaches or surrogate grandparents, and actively join or become part of the family system. The therapists set the tenor of the session. They establish the guidelines for who will talk, when they can talk, and what will or will not be discussed. They make efforts to increase the interpersonal stress either by converting individual problems into family problems or by exposing other problems that have previously not been acknowledged by the family. They also emphasize expanding the family's relationship with the extended family, the culture, and the community; establishing family boundaries; separating the generations; and teaching the family how to play.

SOCIAL LEARNING THEORY

Social learning theory, to which Albert Bandura was a major contributor, is based on behavioral modification, but considered within the context of the family and member interaction. It is designed to teach people how to relate interpersonally within that social environment, and is based on the premise that if appropriate behavioral learning has not been acquired in childhood, people cannot develop adequate social skills. According to Horne (1982), it was first applied to family treatment in the 1960s.

View of the Family

This model views the family as a social system of interacting people. Deviant behavior is seen, not as dysfunction, but as an appropriate response to contingencies of the system.

Major Tenets

The theory postulates continuous reciprocal interaction among cognitive, behavioral, and environmental determinants. It considers that inappropriate behavior is learned through the positive/negative reinforcer trap. Individuals strive to maximize rewards while minimizing costs. Behavior is dealt with either through reinforcement or punishment.

Positive reinforcement involves any action that is presented after an act has been performed and that serves to increase that behavior, whether it is appropriate or inappropriate behavior. For example, praising a child's good behavior, if that behavior increased after the praise, is positive reinforcement. Likewise, encouraging inappropriate conduct because it is funny or otherwise appealing, if that behavior increases following that encouragement, is also positive reinforcement. Negative reinforcement involves removing some stimulus, after an act has been performed, that leads to increased frequency of that act. Taking the privilege of watching television away from a child because he has, for instance, hit his sister, is a negative reinforcer if he then hits his sister even more frequently. If it results in him hitting his sister fewer times, losing television privileges becomes punishment. A reward is merely something given or received in return for doing something, but it is a positive reinforcer only if the rewarded behavior increases.

People tend to think of punishment as doing something to make a child sorry for something he or she has done. However, only if presenting an aversive action or removing a positive action decreases a specific behavior is it punishment. For example, being burned on a hot stove (an aversive stimulus) decreases the frequency of touching a hot stove. Losing driving privileges (a positive stimulus) will likely decrease the frequency of driving offenses. If a behavior increases after a spanking, for instance, the aversive stimulus has become a reinforcer.

This theory contends that social learning takes place within a social environment as a person observes, reacts to, and interacts with other people. Within this social environment, children learn behavior patterns by receiving support for some behaviors and punishment for others.

Goal of Treatment

Treatment aims at providing alternate behaviors to replace the inappropriate behaviors. The therapist presents family members with methods to encourage different responses in their interactions. Parents are taught how to provide appropriate consequences for misbehavior, using a variety of progressive correctional measures.

Therapeutic Style

In this treatment approach, the therapist attempts to provide an environment in which effective learning may occur. Repeated assessment of family interaction is used to evaluate how change is occurring. The focus is on specific identified targeted behaviors and how others in the family are positively or negatively reinforcing the undesirable behavior. The counselor identifies that behavior to be targeted, and gathers baseline data, which is used to plan how to intervene in the behavior. Given the results expected, the therapist may employ a combination of methods such as behavioral contracts, sequenced learning, or extinction.

THE PROCESS MODEL

Virginia Satir (1982) describes her process model as one in which the therapist joins with the family members to move "from a symptomatic base toward one of wellness." Although beginning with individuals, then later with couples, Satir's work evolved into working with families. She considers it necessary to work with the entire family.

View of Family

However well functioning, the family system is balanced and each member "pays a price," whatever the cost, to keep it so. Family rules derive from the way parents maintain their self-esteem and determine how the family system functions. Within this framework, children develop self-esteem. Family problems arise from discrepancies between verbal and nonverbal levels in communication. Satir considers self-esteem to be the central core of communication.

Major Tenets

Satir makes some basic assumptions. The first is that manifested symptoms signal a blockage in an individual's growth and that, however distorted the system may be, family members adapt to the symptom to maintain balance. She further assumes that people have within themselves the resources necessary to grow. The therapist's task is to help them gain access to and use their "nourishing potentials." Moreover, all actions by family members are reciprocal. Satir's fourth assumption is that therapy is an educational process that occurs among individuals. The therapist initiates it by teaching healthy interactions, and directs it toward positive change. Satir defines leveling as the healthy state of communication. Leveling involves having words, body, and feelings all be consistent with the message being conveyed. She has identified four types of individuals with dysfunctional communication styles, as follows.

The *Placater* discounts any sense of self and will behave in a manner to avoid conflict and anger from other people. For this person, worth is based on acceptance by others and being physically available, even when the preference is not to be available. Such people believe their only option is to remain dependent in dysfunctional relationships because they have no choice, have no personal resources, or feel that change is not worth the struggle.

The *Blamer* tends to elevate him- or herself by discounting others and assuming a dominant position to avoid dealing with his or her own issues and responsibilities. Others are blamed for their unhappiness, and they are critical, judgmental, and shaming toward others.

Intellectualizers tend to discount their own feelings. They feel threatened and vulnerable if their feelings are exposed. To avoid experiencing their feelings, they focus on attempts to figure out problems and how to fix them. They are focused on being logical and things making sense to them.

Distracters, to distract and avoid conflict, attempt to turn the focus away from themselves and to others, by being elusive or charming. Their purpose is to keep themselves and others from experiencing painful feelings. Many chemically dependent people master this style of communication, using drugs and alcohol to avoid or deny their problems.

Goal of Treatment

Satir stresses development of individual self-awareness. To experience self, instead of thinking about self, one must work toward becoming healthy. Self-awareness includes the discovery and modification of faulty communication and relationship patterns that hinder healthy functioning.

Therapeutic Style

The therapist joins with the family to promote wellness and functions as a teacher and leader to help people take the risks necessary to take charge of their lives. It is described as a process model because it includes methods and procedures that tend to move the individuals in the family and the family system from symptoms toward wellness. The therapist and the family join forces in this effort. The model may use sculpting to help people totally experience and view themselves objectively. In sculpting, people reexperience previous events by taking physical postures representing the family in that situation. In this way, their communication and relationship patterns can become visible to them. Discrepancies between verbal and non-verbal levels of communication between family members are noted and addressed. Developing a chronology of significant events in people's lives, which Satir refers to as *family reconstruction*, helps identify the origin of various symptoms.

STRUCTURAL FAMILY THERAPY

Colapinto (1982) defines structural family therapy as "a model of treatment based on systems theory." It was developed under the leadership of Salvador Minuchin. A distinctive feature of the model is its emphasis on structure changes as the main goal of therapy, which is considered more important than the details of individual change. Also, the therapist functions as an active agent in restructuring the family.

View of Family

The structural family therapy approach looks at the family as a living, open system with functionally interdependent parts dictated by the overall functioning of the whole. The family's structure is the set of rules by which the members' interactions are regulated. As an open system, the family is subjected to outside influences as well as develops its own structure that extends beyond the family unit. As a living system, the family is constantly being transformed as it faces issues or circumstances that require negotiating the rules by which it functions.

The family maintains its stability and basic characteristics, or homeostasis, by transaction patterns. Change is the adjustment necessary to accommodate to developmental and environmental conditions. The "interplay of homeostasis and change" regulates the family's development. When families cannot make the necessary change, their development stagnates and they avoid conflict, to ensure some sense of balance. Excessive closeness, or enmeshment, at one end of the continuum, and excessive distancing, or disengagement, at the other, are evidence of a high level of conflict avoidance. To maintain their precarious balance, family members adhere to myths that are "very narrow definitions of themselves as a whole and as individuals."

Major Tenets

The structural family therapy approach assumes that families think about and operate within three related areas: the family itself, the presenting problem, and the process of change. Problem behavior is considered within the context of what it is accomplishing for the family and the family's perception of it. Again, this approach emphasizes structural change of the family as the main goal of therapy, with individual change given less importance.

Goal of Treatment

Treatment involves restructuring both the relative positions of family members and the family's system of transactional rules, to permit more flexibility and alternate ways of interacting. To that end, the therapist helps the family establish clearer boundaries and discover hidden conflict.

Therapeutic Style

In this approach, the therapist joins the family system by partially accommodating to the system's rules while maintaining a leadership role. This *joining* provides a format by which dysfunction in the family can be graphically displayed and change can be encouraged. Two techniques employed in joining are *maintenance* and *tracking*. Maintenance involves the therapist becoming "organized by the basic rules that regulate the transaction process in the specific family system." Tracking "consists of an accommodation of the therapist to the content of speech" that is occurring.

The model generally requires working with the entire nuclear family and with as many members of the extended family as possible. The therapist helps family members expose the myths that limit their effective functioning. The therapeutic techniques concurrently challenge while being supportive, attack while being encouraging, and sustain the system while undermining it. Basic to this model is an emphasis on present reality. The focus on a particular individual and the symptom is shifted to the family system and how it reacts to the problem. In other words, a problem does not belong only to one individual but to the entire family.

Interventions designed to change the system involve disequilibration techniques intended to promote a new perspective or create a different sequence of events. *Reframing* is intended to present the problem in a different and more workable manner. *Enactment* seeks to present a new experience to the family that can result in success. *Boundary making* is used to disrupt and modify conflict avoidance patterns and over-involvement of family members. The therapist uses *punctuation* to declare that a transaction has successfully met the therapist's goals. *Unbalancing* describes much of the activity that is occurring by the therapist's attempt to disrupt inappropriate behavior patterns of the family members.

ADLERIAN/DREIKURSIAN FAMILY THERAPY

Lowe (1982) presents ideas and practices that originated with Alfred Adler and Rudolf Dreikurs, as they have been more recently adapted. Initially Adler established a model of individual psychology. His basic concepts included the following: (1) the individual personality "was unified and could be understood only when regarded as a whole," (2) social life for the human being was necessary for survival, which he considered to be a fundamental law of life, (3) there is a natural tendency for human activity to strive "from a feeling of inferiority towards superiority, perfection, totality," and (4) in order to achieve belonging and overcoming, human behavior is goal directed and purposeful.

View of Family

Adlerian concepts applied to family therapy assume that a person's behavior reflects his or her perceived "fit" within the family. Expanding on Adler's perception of goal-directed behavior, Dreikurs identified four goals of a child's disruptive behavior. He considered that to find a place in the group, "every action of a child has a purpose." The well-adjusted child, by conforming and contributing to family norms, has found social acceptance. The misbehaving child, in an attempt to gain the social acceptance that he believes he is missing, will "(1) try to get attention or (2) attempt to prove his power, or (3) he may seek revenge or (4) display his deficiency in order to get special service or exemption." This theoretical view is the basis for principles of child-rearing and parenting practices widely used in recent years.

Major Tenets

Adlerian theory holds that the personality is unified and can be understood only when regarded as a whole. Human beings are social animals and need to belong. The one basic dynamic force behind all human behavior is a striving to overcome inferiority. All behavior is goal directed and purposeful. A major focus is the child's goals and motivation as they relate to the child finding a place in the group and how adults encourage or discourage the child's behavior in doing so. The misbehaving child bases his or her behavior on a conviction that this is the only way he or she can function within the family.

In learning to make decisions and to assume responsibility, children need a stable environment in which to be able to predict outcomes. Dreikurs contends that, rather than parental punishment, allowing children to suffer the natural and logical consequences of their maladaptive behavior is the best way to correct it. Scolding, humiliation, reprimands, and punishment only add to the discouragement that the misbehaving child has already internalized and deprive the child of the ability to learn more responsibility. Praise and rewards rendered only for acceptable behavior convey the message that in exchange for certain approved kinds of behavior the child will be highly valued. Therefore, with less approved behavior the child will be less valued. In other words, the value or acceptance of the child is based solely on performance and behavior. Encouragement, in contrast, has the potential for assuring that parents have confidence in the child and conveys the message that the child is highly valued whatever the behavior might be. Showing enthusiasm for a child's participation in an event, whether he or she excels or not, helping the child overcome some difficulty in performing a task, or thanking him or her for the effort put forth, are ways to provide encouragement.

Goal of Treatment

The primary goal of treatment is to gain the skills necessary to improve the parent–child relationship. This initially entails helping the parents understand the poor dynamics involved. Then the parents can develop alternative ways to deal with the child's behavior, and to gain the courage to take risks in finding viable resolutions for the child's misbehavior.

Therapeutic Style

The primary focus is on the locus of complaint or the individual identified as the problem, and on using encouragement to alter behavior and create a personal internal locus of control. The therapist helps the parents identify the intent or purposefulness of the child's behavior and to develop contingencies with which to encourage change in behavior.

TRANSACTIONAL ANALYSIS

Richard Erskine (1982) outlines the fundamentals of Transactional Analysis. TA was originated by Eric Berne (1964) to provide a framework for analyzing transactions among people as well as the transactions, or self-talk, within a single person. Berne contends that transactions occur among three ego states: Parent, Adult, and Child.

The Parent ego state is the part of the personality where we reexperience what we imagined were our own parents' feelings in a particular situation, or where we feel and act toward others as our parents felt and acted toward us. The Nurturing Parent is consoling, empathic, and caring. The Critical Parent imposes "shoulds" and "musts." It conveys the message that something was done wrong, could have been done better, or shouldn't be done at all.

The Adult ego state is the objective part of the personality, or the data processor. It is neither emotional nor judgmental. It interacts with others on a mature, nonemotional, and rational basis.

The Child ego state consists of feelings, impulses, and spontaneous acts. This state represents the Natural Child as being the impulsive, untrained, spontaneous, expressive infant in each of us. The Little Professor is the natural wisdom of a child, which is manipulative, egocentric, creative, and intuitive. The Adapted Child exhibits modifications of the Natural Child's inclinations as the result of traumatic experiences, demands, training, and decisions about how to get attention. It whines, complies, or rebels.

View of Family

TA embraces and integrates several concepts regarding the family. Children grow up with parental injunctions, and on the basis of these messages they make their early decisions. An injunction is a message, direct or implied, given to the child from a parent's internal child, which originates in his or her own pain, anxiety, anger, frustration, and unhappiness. These messages tell children what they must do and be to get recognition. The injunctions tell the child, "Don't"—"Don't be, don't be close, don't be important, don't be a child, don't grow, don't succeed, don't be you, don't be sane, or don't belong."

Children decide either to accept or fight against these parental messages. If certain injunctions are accepted, the early decision is then made to incorporate that belief into the basic part of a permanent character structure. Many of the injunctions may have been appropriate in certain situations in childhood, but they are carried over and generalized into adulthood.

The early decisions children make are aimed at receiving recognition and attention, or parental strokes. Parents express strokes in physical touch, words, and gestures. Positive strokes convey, "I like you," and negative strokes say, "I don't like you." Conditional strokes impart the message, "I will like you if and when you are or behave in a certain way." Unconditional strokes convey the message, "I am willing to accept you for who you are and for being who you are, and we can negotiate our differences."

Major Tenets

Transactional analysis is antideterministic in that it contends that people are capable of transcending their conditioning and early childhood programming. It acknowledges that early childhood influences play an important role in human development, but believes that decisions about life choices can be reviewed, challenged, and changed. The ego state from which one functions may vary with different relationships. As people become more aware of the ego state in which they are operating, they also can become more aware of their adaptive behavior and become better able to choose other options.

Once early childhood decisions are made, says Berne, *games* are developed to support those original decisions and become part of a person's *life script*. A game is an ongoing series of transactions that ends with a bad feeling for at least one of the players. By their very nature, games are designed to prevent intimacy.

The familiar unpleasant feelings experienced after a game are called *rackets*. The person often experienced these feelings with his or her parents, and held on to and saved them up. Rackets also support early decisions and become a basic part of one's life script. Whether they involve anger, guilt, or depression, rackets are maintained by actually choosing situations that will support unpleasant and chronic feelings.

All these elements fit into the *life script*, which includes the person's expectations of how his or her life drama will be played out. It includes the parental messages that the person has incorporated and the decisions the person has made in response to these injunctions. The life script also incorporates the games played to maintain the early decisions, the rackets experienced to justify decisions, and the expectations of the way one thinks his or her life drama will be played out and how the story will end.

Goal of Treatment
The basic goal of transactional analysis is to help clients make new decisions about their present behavior and the direction of their lives. The goal is for clients to gain awareness of how they have restricted their freedom of choice by following early decisions about their life positions. Therapists teach people to write their own scripts instead of being passively scripted by the past.

Therapeutic Style
In TA, the counselor functions as a teacher of and partner with the client. Specific techniques include role-playing, empty-chair work, family modeling, and analyzing rituals, pastimes, games, rackets, and scripts.

FAMILY SYSTEMS THEORY

Murray Bowen's family systems theory developed from his many years of experience with families, beginning with his work with schizophrenics. The theory is based on the premise that family emotional and living patterns cross multiple generations. It provides a basis of looking at families from that perspective. Addressing the emotional intensity and the challenges that can abound in working with families in chaos, Bowen places a great deal of emphasis on therapists having a strong foundation in theory. Without such theory, the therapist, particularly a novice, can easily lose emotional self-control and become engulfed in the family's emotional system. Bowen saw schizophrenia as an extreme symptom of fusion within an undifferentiated family system. He considered schizophrenia to be a product of a multigenerational decline in differentiation over at least eight to ten generations.

View of the Family
Bowen (1978) views the family as a network or system composed of not only the members of the nuclear family, but also the extended families.

All members of the family operate within an emotional force that is essential to maintain the system's homeostasis, or equilibrium. For that reason, the therapist considers the functioning of the entire family, even if working only with a single person.

Major Tenets

The family systems approach contends that people and families function on a continuum, often in imbalance, between differentiation and fusion. Bowen considers that the family's symptoms are a way to deal with the tension of fusion. Using the perspective of dealing with the family's emotional intensity, Bowen developed eight concepts:

1. *Differentiation of self/fusion.* It is from this concept that Bowen formulated his other concepts. His past research with schizophrenics revealed a reciprocal mother–child emotional relationship that he labeled *symbiosis.* From later findings he concluded that the symbiosis also involved the father and other siblings. This broader relationship he labeled **fusion.** The polar opposite of fusion is **differentiation of self.**
2. *Triangles.* Family triangles describe the process of fusion between two people who incorporate a third party to relieve anxiety the two are experiencing.
3. *Nuclear family emotional system.* The nuclear emotional system consists of the patterns of the family's emotional functioning within a single generation.
4. *Family projection process.* This is an extension of the fusion that involves projection of the problem to the other members of the triangle.
5. *Emotional cutoff.* Basically, emotional cutoff is the denial of the unresolved emotional attachment to the previous generation.
6. *Multigenerational transmission process.* In the **multigenerational transmission process,** levels of functioning are carried from one generation to succeeding generations.
7. *Sibling positions.* Bowen considers that the sibling positions are an important factor in developing family roles.
8. *The process in society.* This final concept refers to Bowen's contention that interactions similar to the family's can be seen in society as a whole due to the "imbalance between population size and the availability of natural resources."

Succeeding chapters address the first six of these concepts further.

Goal of Treatment

The primary goal of treatment is to help each family member to achieve a higher level of self differentiation. Accomplishing that goal requires detriangulating and resolving those issues that resulted in emotional cutoff from the extended family. Detriangulation involves becoming emotionally unhooked from the system.

Therapeutic Style

This theory takes a historical approach by uncovering multigenerational patterns of interaction. The family systems approach defines therapy more in terms of a philosophical approach rather than any particular technique. By uncovering those patterns that have persisted as maladaptive functioning, the therapist hopes to direct the family members to modifying their roles, boundaries, and interactions. The therapist often works with only those members of the family who prove the most motivated to change, rather than the entire family. The rationale is that if one or two members of the family can make significant changes in role and boundary definition, the other members automatically have to adapt their functioning.

CONCLUSION

It is important to note that the techniques used in any one therapeutic style are not necessarily better than those used in another, nor need using any one style necessarily exclude using others as well. Different approaches and techniques may be effective with different people and in different applications. However, I believe the therapist should have a solid theoretical foundation in whichever therapeutic approach best fits with his or her personal philosophy, training, and personality, rather than just grasping at little bits and pieces of several.

Family systems theory has emerged from the child guidance, marital counseling, and social work fields and provides a concrete method of observing and understanding family dynamics. From my observation, it encompasses the theoretical premise from which the dynamics involved within the chemically dependent family can most aptly be defined and treated.

Chapter Four

The Family as a System

To adequately understand families, the individual members' behavior must be examined within the context of the family system. In addition, most family theorists agree that the individual member's problematic behavior is an outcome of family interactions within that system and not exclusively of individual dynamics.

A system, as defined in The American Heritage Dictionary (New College edition), is "a group of interacting, interrelated, or inter-dependent elements forming or regarded as forming a collective entity." Thus an interdependent element is capable both of functioning separately and in reliance on and influenced by the interrelated interaction or functioning of other elements within the system. As a system, therefore, the functioning of the family (the collective entity) is determined by the way in which the individual family members (the interdependent elements) interact and interrelate. When A causes event B, causality is linear. However, in a system context, causality is circular or reciprocal. That is, A affects B and C and D as much as each of them in turn affect A.

Virginia Satir (1967) was probably the person who first compared the family system to a mobile. The family system as just defined can likewise be compared to a mobile. The pieces all connect in some fashion. Each piece is independent to the extent that as the mobile hangs in balance, or homeostasis, one piece does not touch another. However, when a breeze comes along, the individual pieces are all shown to be interdependent, because whichever way one piece moves it influences the other pieces to move as well. When the breeze ceases, the mobile pieces gradually return to homeostasis, which exemplifies a healthy family. In an unhealthy family the various pieces, or members, tend to become entangled with each other so that they are unable to function independently.

In family systems theory (Kerr & Bowen, 1988), the factor that most influences the functioning of families and its members is its pattern or style of living and interacting. This pattern is "inherited" from respective families of origin, defined by Bowen as the multigenerational transmission process. Simply stated, people learn to communicate, to relate and interact with others, to love, to parent, and to function from patterns developed and nurtured by their own parents, who acquired them from previous generations.

The individual accommodation to and perpetual reenactment of these living generational patterns grounds the dynamics of families in which chemical dependency exists. Many workers in the chemical dependency field accept that there is a genetic, biological predisposition to addiction. However, according to Steinglass (1987), the family's interactional patterns determine its attitudes about alcohol and drug use and how that use is or is not to be accepted and dealt with as a family problem.

THE FAMILY EMOTIONAL SYSTEM

Kerr and Bowen (1988) describe the emotional system of a family "as the existence of a naturally occurring system in all forms of life that enables an organism to receive information both from within itself and from the environment, to integrate that information, and to respond on the basis of that information" (p. 27). Stated simply, how the person thinks about, or cognitively processes information, determines his or her associated feelings. Conversely, how a person feels about the information received determines what he or she thinks about it. Individuals function within the family system in cognitive/emotional states. Because cognition and emotion are interdependent, families develop systems of patterned emotional functioning. These patterns are based on both instinctual responses and learned factors.

The emotional functioning of individual family members generates a family atmosphere that in turn influences the emotional functioning of each person. Within this emotional system, people respond sometimes based on their own self-interest and sometimes on the broader interests of the group. The intensity of this emotional atmosphere varies from family to family.

The family emotional atmosphere significantly influences individual beliefs, values, attitudes, feelings, and behavior. People occupy different functioning positions in this emotional system or atmosphere. These functions operate reciprocally and influence interactions and behavior within the family. The actions of one member shape the behavior of the other members as well as the family emotional system itself.

The parents who establish the rules, patterns, interactions, and decision-making styles create the general family atmosphere. The locus of control generally lies with the most dysfunctional member of the family—in the chemically dependent family, most often with the dependent person. However, the most dysfunctional member may not necessarily be the addicted person. The functioning of another family member in reaction to the chemically dependent may be the most dysfunctional. In that case, that other person commands the locus of control.

Every family has varying degrees of competition and cooperation among its members. However, based on each individual's perceived reality, the family atmosphere is often interpreted differently by each member of the family. For example, one person might view the addiction of a member as being intrusive, whereas, simultaneously, another sees it as a norm.

Bowen observed that people tend to develop a level of **emotional maturity** dependent on maturity of their parents, and of their grandparents. He refers to this maturity level as the *level of differentiation*. To the extent that the concept describes an individual's level of functioning, terms with similar meanings used by other theorists are *individuality*, *authenticity*, and *emotional maturity*. The exact definition of these terms may vary somewhat from one theorist to another, but the general intent is comparable. A person demonstrates differentiation of self by the ability to be fully functional apart from an emotional connection with another person. In other words, a differentiated person is not emotionally dependent on another individual or individuals.

Although I adhere to Bowen's concept of differentiation of self, I tend to use the term *emotional maturity* when referring to levels of differentiation, or individual functioning, and *differentiation* when referring to the degree of separation from the extended family (addressed later). This separation in definition seems to be easier to grasp for my students and clients.

According to Kerr and Bowen (1988), within the family system, at any point in time, the level of functioning depends on four factors: (1) the basic level of emotional maturity (or differentiation) of its members, (2) the level of stress, (3) the patterns of symptomatic reaction peculiar to the family or a particular family member, and (4) the level of adult-to-adult contact with members of the extended family. A grown child still intent on living up to parental expectations, or seeking parental approval, is operating at the level of child-to-adult rather than adult-to-adult.

OVER- AND UNDERRESPONSIBILITY

Most families have a member or members who function overresponsibly at least in response to certain specific situations, if not in most areas of family activity. However, the extent to which this occurs depends on the family's level of emotional maturity. The **overresponsible person** typically feels responsible for the emotional well-being of others. This individual tries to compensate for any real or perceived deficits in the functioning of others, particularly of those considered to be under-responsible. This role gives that person a way to derive strength and confidence from the dependency of others and to establish or maintain control. In the most severe cases of overresponsibility, the person maintains control by whatever seems most effective, and very often at all costs. The person may manifest control by making decisions for others, doing "what's best" for others, or using various tactics of manipulation. This effort of control is often made with the intent or in the guise of protecting other family members from some consequence. In the chemically dependent family, the overresponsible member often takes on an enabling role by attempting to cover up drinking/drug use actions, and/or making excuses to the dependent's employer, family, and friends.

The **underresponsible person** tends to give up too much self-control and too much self. That person becomes more and more dependent on the overresponsible one. Ultimately the person loses all sense of self and self-confidence. According to Kerr and Bowen (1988), it is generally much easier for family members to accommodate to and make allowances for the underfunctioning person than to address the underlying relationship. In the chemically dependent family, accommodation may occur to avoid actually dealing with the drinking/drug use. An example is the overresponsible wife who sets the alarm to awaken her so that she can make sure her underresponsible husband gets up and ready for work on a morning after he has been drinking heavily.

INDIVIDUALITY AND TOGETHERNESS

The most fundamental characteristic of a person's emotional system is that it operates as if governed by the interplay of two counterbalancing forces that Kerr and Bowen (1988) describe as *individuality* and *togetherness.*

The drive for individuality leads a person to follow his or her own directives and to be an independent and distinct entity. Individuality allows one to feel, think, and act for oneself without concern about whether others approve or in deference to how others feel, think, and act. The person largely motivated by individuality develops a self-identity that says, "I am who I am with or without another." In a family where individuality exists, members are able to communicate effectively with each other and to function in a healthy manner both within and outside the unit.

In contrast, togetherness propels a person to follow the directives of others and to be a dependent, connected, and indistinct entity. This drive is reflected in the need for approval and to act, feel, and think like others. It also carries the expectation that others act, feel, and think the same.

The person dominated by togetherness develops a self-identity based solely on the relationship with another. Such a personality says, "I can't exist, or am nothing, outside this relationship." A family with strong togetherness needs becomes enmeshed. Enmeshment blocks the members from being able to communicate effectively with others and to function in a healthy manner.

Any emotionally significant relationship, to develop, must find a state of balance. Balance is achieved through the interplay between individuality and togetherness. A person tends to gravitate toward someone who is willing to make an equal investment of energy to the relationship. It is often said that opposites attract, and this is often true, but doesn't necessarily create a healthy relationship. Two individuals at a fairly equal and higher level of emotional maturity achieve a healthy balance. In such a relationship, togetherness is less intense, emotional reactiveness is better regulated, and only a low level of energy investment is required. The partners feel a basic attraction and interest in each other rather than one or both being consumed with deep yearnings and needs.

The pairing of two individuals with low levels of emotional maturity achieves an unhealthy balance. Such a relationship requires a high level of energy investment. For example, an overresponsible individual paired with an underresponsible individual forms a **complementarity** that requires much energy to maintain. A person who takes on responsibility for the well-being of another has as little ability to direct his or her life separate from the relationship as does the dependent person. Kerr and Bowen (1988) demonstrate the effect of the various levels of emotional maturity and the amount of energy required in the togetherness force, in Figures 4-1 through 4-4.

The large shaded area in Figure 4-1 represents a relationship with very low levels of emotional maturity, a high degree of togetherness, or enmeshment; and a very high level of energy. Each person's functioning is directly influenced by and dependent on the other and the relationship itself. Neither person has the capacity for autonomous functioning. Each person's functioning becomes totally governed by what transpires between the two of them. The parties are so responsive to signals from the other, and the emotional reactiveness is so intense, that they virtually become prisoners of the relationship. If not actively involved in a significant relationship, the person has considerable difficulty managing his or her life and achieving emotional well-being.

Figure 4-2 represents people with slightly higher levels of emotional maturity and a somewhat lower energy level in the relationship. They have some capacity for autonomous functioning, but are still barely emotionally developed. The relationship provides a sense of complete-ness, an identity, and a greater sense of personal self-worth for the partners. As a result, individual functioning can vacillate from being

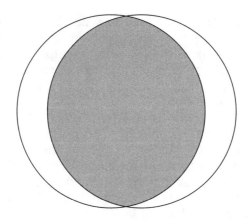

FIGURE 4-1 _____

unable to function at all to being markedly enhanced by the relationship. Although a fraction of autonomous functioning can be retained in the relationship, for the most part individual functioning is governed by the relationship itself. If the people are not actively involved in a relationship, they can barely attain a sense of individual completeness and emotional well-being.

People possessing yet greater individual autonomous functioning, as suggested in Figure 4-3, become less automatically governed by and dependent on the relationship. Each partner is somewhat complete, and can be fairly autonomous in the relationship without continually needing emotional reinforcement. The relationship, therefore, requires lesser energy. If not involved in a relationship, the individuals can manage their lives effectively and retain some sense of emotional well-being.

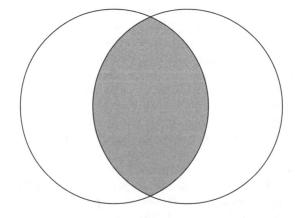

FIGURE 4-2 _____

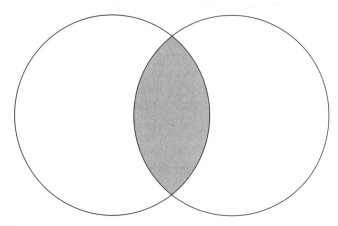

FIGURE 4-3 _____

Figure 4-4 depicts a relationship of highly emotionally developed people. They can be actively involved in a relationship and yet remain self-determined and autonomous. Each can respond to input from the other on a feeling and subjective level, but can process these responses on an objective level. This eliminates automatic emotional reactiveness and permits choice. The need for togetherness is minimal, and although each is attracted to and interested in the other, their functioning does not depend on each other's presence, acceptance, or approval. Their expectations of each other are governed by the realities of cooperation rather than by some infantile need. This degree of individual self-containment means that the relationship has little anxiety.

People in a dependent relationship tend to feed off one another. This can be depicted as shown in Figure 4-5; the entire emotional process of a dependent person is circuitous.

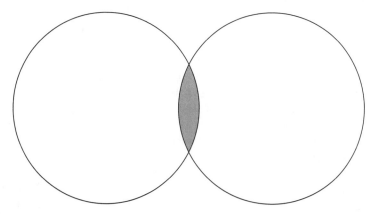

FIGURE 4-4 _____

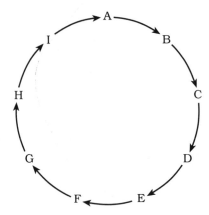

***FIGURE* 4-5** _____

The lower the individual level of emotional maturity (A), the greater the **emotional dependency** in a relationship (B) and the more easily threatened the parties become (C). The more threatened they feel, the more intense their anxiety (D). The more anxiety they experience, the more energy they invest in actions or behaviors designed to reduce that anxiety (E) and the more the boundaries between the parties become diffused (F). As the boundaries dissolve, the partners become even more reactive to each other's distress and use more energy to avoid saying or doing things that will increase disapproval or conflict (G). The conflict avoidance is an attempt to enhance another's emotional well-being. Unfortunately, it only creates a situation of "walking on eggshells" to not trigger an upset in the relationship. Consequently, the increased anxiety pressures the parties to adapt to each other in whatever manner will reduce the anxiety (H). As the people make adaptations or accommodations to avoid pressure created by anxiety, they devote even less energy to being an individual (I), while focusing on and responding to the other, with a resultant further loss of self (A), thus continuing the cycle.

Excessive adaptation to preserve harmony in the relationship leads to a sacrifice of self and to feeling not in control of personal functioning. Such a person is convinced that his or her well-being depends on the way others respond to him or her. In such relationships, a person may attempt to gain or regain personal control with a number of direct or manipulative behaviors. The partners may also show one or more symptoms such as an eating disorder, excessive drug or alcohol use, depression, or other compulsive behaviors. Over- or underachieving becomes a way to get attention through praise or criticism. Other people might begin an affair, or even develop physical problems. Under these circumstances, the partners usually feel trapped in the relationship, because they cannot imagine solutions to the problems or a way out of the dysfunction.

Even if someone leaves the relationship, the high level of neediness and anxiety of emotionally dependent people persist. Consequently, when the anxiety with the relationship becomes too intense, people may become what Steinglass (1987) refers to as "relationship nomads." That is they are continually changing relationships, always seeking the "perfect" mate. Because the original living patterns that resulted in the relationship-related anxiety are still there, future relationships will have similar difficulties. Encountering consistent high levels of anxiety may eventually result in such people avoiding relationships altogether.

In almost any relationship, the partners do not always want the same amount of closeness or distancing. Emotionally mature people can accept this without emotional reactiveness and interpret the discrepancy perhaps only as a slight disappointment or an inconvenience. In emotionally immature relationships with a high level of emotional dependency, one partner can interpret the other's lack of responsiveness as something wrong, as personal rejection or lack of love. This interpretation can create a lot of conflict and anxiety in the relationship.

When an intense need for togetherness exists, people seem addicted to each other. Each tends to make presumptions about the other based on his or her own beliefs and feelings. Although they may feel an occasional urge to escape each other, neither has the capacity to do so. This relationship addiction can feel just as physical as addiction to a drug. A person's sense of emotional well-being becomes dependent on how that person perceives him- or herself to be loved, thought about, and responded to by the other.

The emotional maturity of the parties determines how the emergence of critical issues such as chemical dependency affect the relationship. (This can be true of issues such as mental disorder or physical impairment as well.) The highly mature family usually experiences a temporary adjustment period to make any necessary adaptations after a crisis, and then restabilize. In families with very low levels of maturity, however, the relationship process may develop around the identified patient, such as the alcoholic member.

According to Steinglass (1987), the family's focus on the problems of one person, such as the alcoholic, may create a type of togetherness that in itself becomes fairly stable. Taking care of or protecting the identified patient can become self-satisfying itself or provide a sense of meaning to one's life. In other words, the family establishes a balance around the dysfunction created by the addiction. The family finds it easier to live with a chronic symptom or dysfunction than to confront the basic relationship problems. The symptom tends to take the focus off the problems created by the family's emotional immaturity and faulty interaction patterns.

To further complicate family emotional development, the chemically dependent person generally has an arrested emotional maturation, particularly if regular usage began at a young age. This person has sacrificed normal developmental tasks of achieving a healthy sense of self or of personal identity. The alcohol or drugs have substituted for the development of self-esteem, confidence, and effective communication skills, leaving the individual with a sense of insecurity.

EXERCISES

1. Give and analyze three examples of (a) how a person's thinking determines associated feelings and (b) how a person's feelings about a situation determine associated thoughts.
2. Provide and discuss three examples of emotional responses based on (a) self-interest, and three based on (b) the broader interests of the family.
3. Describe three situations that may occur within families, and identify the locus of control in each.
4. Describe three examples of complementarity, or over- and under-responsibility.
5. Describe a family interaction that suggests enmeshment.
6. Give three examples of accommodation to the underresponsible member of a chemically dependent family.

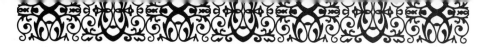

Chapter Five

Elements of the Emotional System

As previously defined, a system is "a group of interacting, interrelated, or interdependent elements forming or regarded as forming a collective entity." So of course a family emotional system also contains basic elements or components that require consideration.

SYMBIOSIS

In his work with schizophrenics and their families, Murray Bowen (1988) discovered that hospital staff reported some interesting occurrences among family members. As a patient began to improve, members of the patient's family would complain either that they had observed worsening symptoms or that someone else in the family had become ill or dysfunctional. Bowen also observed a reciprocal emotional interaction between the mother and patient that he labeled the mother–child symbiosis. Bowen concluded that some kind of a powerful emotional force worked within the family system to maintain a balance of conflicting forces.

Symbiosis, as described by Bowen, is a two-person system in which responsible individuality does not nor cannot develop. It is as if each person lives only for and vicariously through the other. Each person in the symbiotic relationship seems compelled to ensure, at any cost, the other person's emotional comfort. One person can only be comfortable and happy when the other is comfortable and happy. They sacrifice all their personal goals and self needs to ensure short-term peace and harmony.

In a symbiotic relationship, any attention or attempt of one of the partners directed away from the other and toward someone outside the relationship is likely to be viewed by the other with extreme jealousy or a feeling of rejection. They may expect that any chosen activity should include both parties. Any attempt by one to be involved in some activity without the other may be met with faked illness, accusations of not being appreciated, or some subterfuge to disable the plans. To maintain stability in the relationship, even insignificant decisions by one are likely not to be made without the approval of the other. For example, a mother in a symbiotic relationship with her daughter devotes a considerable amount of energy to maintaining that relationship. The mother may consider the relationship between her and her daughter as that of best friends, and may resent the daughter's attempt to acquire friends of her own. The mother may accuse the daughter of not appreciating all that has been done for her.

Although a symbiotic relationship is most often noted between mother and child, it can also exist between others. One couple with which I worked some years ago, both alcoholic, was an extreme example of this kind of relationship. Everything one did had to include the other. They excluded other people, including members of their extended families, from sharing any of their time together. The wife accompanied her husband daily on his delivery job. Their children were often neglected because they interfered too much in the couple's togetherness. As a result, the children were eventually placed in foster care. Both parents said they loved their children and wanted to regain custody. However, they were more concerned about preserving their status quo than in making the necessary changes. As a result, neither of them were able to achieve any degree of recovery because they were so emotionally dependent on each other.

At some point, one or both participants in a symbiotic relationship become frustrated or angry at having to sacrifice so much for the relationship, particularly if they begin to feel they're not getting enough in return for their sacrifices. Tension surfaces and attempts at harmony fail. When tension begins to surface, it then incorporates a wider relationship, in a process that Bowen calls *fusion*. This wider relationship may now involve the other parent, or other siblings or, in the case of a married couple, someone outside the immediate family. When this fusion with another person occurs, the symbiotic relationship changes from a dyad to a triangle.

TRIANGULATION

Kerr and Bowen (1988) consider the triangle to be the basic molecule of *fan* an emotional system. The dynamics of a triangle preserve equilibrium in the three-party system. As long as anxiety remains low, a two-person system can remain fairly calm and stable. As tension or anxiety increases, however, a third person is drawn in and becomes involved in the tension of the twosome. The added third person creates the triangle. The involvement of the third person decreases the anxiety in the twosome by allowing tension to be shifted around the triangle. This reduces the possibility of any one relationship emotionally overheating or erupting. According to Bowen, triangles exist in all families to some extent, but may

dyad

never become symptomatic. Almost every family has one child who is more triangulated than the others and whose life adjustment is not as good as that of the other siblings.

Because tension can be shifted around, the triangle offers more flexibility than does the two-person relationship (Figure 5-1). Unfortunately, within the triangle a two-against-one dynamic often appears. The third person (C) who completes the triangle may be expected to resolve, or may be held responsible for, the problems between A and B. Most often a poorly differentiated child occupies this position with a parent. For example, a daughter (B) in a symbiotic relationship with her mother (A) may begin to rebel against the mother's control over her life and present some kind of problem or behavior. When the tension reaches a certain level, the mother may draw in the father (C) to help control the daughter. With both parents focusing on the child, the conflict between mother and daughter can be temporarily set aside.

Bowen further describes triangles as having a basic character with which to stabilize or destabilize a twosome. A stable twosome can be destabilized by the addition or removal of a third person. Conversely, an unstable twosome can be stabilized by the addition or removal of the third person. The third person may be a new baby, or a child who leaves home. For example, if the conflict between the marital partners ceases following the entry or departure of the child, the change has had a stabilizing effect. If conflict arises in a harmonious couple after the addition or departure of the child, the change has had a destabilizing effect.

The emotional circuitry of a triangle, once established, is usually perpetuated by involving others. In other words, if one person of the triangle dies or leaves, another person will, because family stabilization requires it, step in to fill the vacancy. Because children often act out

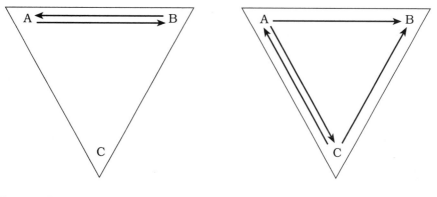

FIGURE 5-1

conflict that was never resolved between their parents, the triangulation can continue into succeeding generations.

The more enmeshed a family, the more triangulation is necessary to ensure some sense of emotional stability in the system. The family can contain tension within the triangle as long as they can shift it around the three sides. However, when the tension of the triangle becomes high enough, it spills over to pick up a vulnerable fourth person (Figure 5-2). That person's participation then adds one or more new triangles, thus forming a small network of triangles, or what Bowen refers to as interlocking triangles. For example, mother (A) and daughter Judy (B) of the triangle get into conflict over appropriate dress and older sister Sue (C) temporarily withdraws from the triangle. The mother (A) pulls in the father (D) to help settle the dispute with Judy, while Sue engages in another triangle with the father and the brother.

This process can continue until personal triangles within the family have been exhausted and the tension then spills over into the public arena, involving police, social workers, and counselors. A really successful extension of the triangulation process has occurred, for example, when outside social workers are arguing with each other about individual or family treatment needs or consequences to be imposed on one family member (Figure 5-3). In the meantime, the family becomes calmer and more united because the pressure has been taken off of them.

A common triangle that might exist is between an adult child and the parents. Suppose, for example, that every time Jane visits her parents, the mother takes her aside and starts complaining about the father. Jane may feel good about being taken into her mother's confidence and may even feel she can help her parents resolve their problems. But in fact, this alliance with the mother is destructive to all three relationships: Jane and father, father and mother, and Jane and mother. Siding with her mother alienates her father. It also makes it less likely that the mother

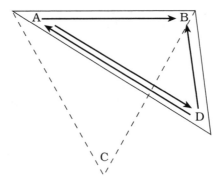

FIGURE 5-2

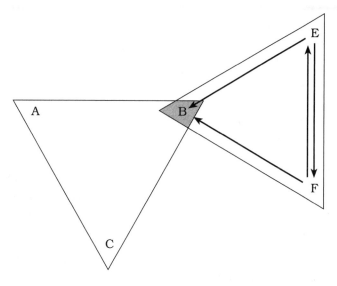

FIGURE 5-3

will do anything about working out her problems with the father. Although this triangle may give the illusion that Jane is close to her mother, it is at best only an imitation of intimacy. Nor would Jane's defense of her father be a solution. That would only move her away from her mother and would widen the gulf between mother and father. As long as the triangulation continues among the three parties, a personal and open one-to-one relationship cannot develop. The simplest and most direct approach to this situation would be for Jane to suggest that mother and father work out the problem between themselves, and to refuse to become involved or even allow the mother to confide in her.

The functioning positions of members in a triangle can be fairly rigid and somewhat predictable. Bowen describes them in relation to the anxiety being experienced. The *anxiety generator* is the first person in the triangle to become anxious about the situation and is often held responsible for initiating the upsets. The *anxiety amplifier* adds to the problem by reacting in an agitated and exaggerated manner to the anxiety of the generator. The *anxiety dampener* remains emotionally distanced in reaction to the problem until the tension is great enough that he or she will become overly responsible in an attempt to calm the others down. Although the tension may be reduced temporarily in this scenario, the problem remains unsolved. The dampener only further reinforces the triangle, and no one takes responsibility for managing his or her own anxiety.

For one person to attain emotional separation, or differentiation, from such a family, **detriangulation** must occur. Effective detriangling depends on one person achieving some degree of emotional **detachment** from and emotional neutrality regarding the family. The person must communicate the position of emotional neutrality to the rest of the family, and must change his or her basic way of responding to family problems. Emotional neutrality doesn't mean that one becomes indifferent to or judgmental of other family members' problems. It must, however, involve a conviction that finding a solution for the problems of others is their responsibility, even if they don't seem to be "doing it right." Assuming an attitude of "people have a right to be wrong" can help one remain neutral.

Detriangling is not an easy process, and takes time, practice, and experience. Other family members often become so threatened by one person's attempt to detriangle and seek emotional separation that they impose consequences. The family's imposed consequence might be to give the defector the silent treatment, accuse the person of being disloyal to the family, or even completely exclude that person from the family. A prevailing attitude among the other family members involved in the triangulation is often "If you're not with us, you're against us."

EMOTIONAL MATURITY (SELF-DIFFERENTIATION)

Bowen considers self-differentiation as a person's ability to adapt to stress and to distinguish between the processes of feeling and intellect. In other words, the degree of self-differentiation is the degree to which one can choose between being guided by feelings or thoughts, and being engulfed in the emotional problems of others. Self-differentiation has nothing to do with intelligence or educational level, only the degree to which a person is emotionally mature and can function independently in life.

The level of emotional maturity at which one functions lies on a continuum from very poor to high. At the lower end of the continuum, people experience a high level of chronic anxiety. They are emotionally needy and highly reactive to the actions and feelings of others. They have difficulty maintaining long-term relationships and cannot differentiate between thoughts and feelings. They tend to make assumptions about what is right for others and to become triangulated with them. Their daily functioning is almost totally governed by their emotional reactions to others. The self is so poorly developed that they experience love primarily as neediness, and attain a sense of completeness only with an emotional attachment to another. The person is not separated from the family of origin, and such a person often remains in an unsatisfactory relationship because "it's better than nothing."

At the opposite end of the continuum, the emotionally mature person can think objectively about emotionally sensitive issues yet can respond appropriately rather than simply react. The person can communicate needs and wants openly without emotional reactivity. He or she assumes responsibility for self as well as for his or her own feelings and happiness. Such a person can function without being affected by praise or criticism, and has the freedom to enjoy rather than just need relationships. He or she experiences inner security and a low level of anxiety.

The basic level of emotional maturity is fairly well established by the time a child reaches adolescence and usually remains fixed for life. Change may occur because the person has an unusual life experience or tires of a dysfunctional lifestyle, which may force the person to make a focused effort to raise his or her functioning level. However, the odds of people at the extreme low end of the continuum even making the effort to change are not very favorable. If they seek to improve their life situation and happiness, the attempt will likely amount to efforts to find someone to "fix" them or to "fix" another person involved in the situation.

I have had many clients, both men and women, who come into counseling because their relationship has dissolved and they cannot adjust to aloneness. They have become so preoccupied with the misery of being apart and lonely that they cannot function adequately. Some are so incapacitated that they cannot perform their jobs adequately. Such a person's sense of completeness is based solely on being in the relationship. It is not unusual for the breakup to be only temporary, and this person may even return to an abusive relationship. Or they may shift their expression of undying love to another person who may come along. If either of those events occur, they will stop therapy, because they perceive their life as being all right again.

Most people want to be individuals, but are not emotionally developed enough to give up togetherness to achieve more individuality. People are often willing to be individuals only to the extent that the existing relationship system approves and permits it. Anything else is considered too risky for the relationship. For instance, a woman may have someone she considers to be a very good friend, but will give up the friendship because the man she's currently involved with either disapproves of the friend or is jealous of time spent with her. But for mature people, giving up togetherness does not mean giving up emotional closeness. It does mean that one's functioning becomes less dependent on the approval and acceptance of others.

Possessing emotional maturity is a way of being, of living, or of experiencing life. The better developed the self, the more a person can act to enhance his or her personal welfare without impinging on the welfare of others. Conversely, a lack of emotional maturity, and the need for togetherness, result in partners encroaching on one another and functioning at one another's expense. In an emotionally healthy or well-differentiated system, people can maintain their emotional autonomy. In such a system triangulation is minimal, because the system's stability does not depend on it.

DEVELOPMENTAL FACTORS

Every human being enters the world totally dependent on others for survival and comfort. In most instances, this dependency rests on the primary caretaker, the mother. Because of this total dependence and because mother and infant respond so automatically to one another, Bowen considers the symbiotic relationship to develop naturally. However, as the child grows, a series of age-specific developmental tasks must be accomplished for that child to become a unique individual and to develop individuality and emotional maturity. As long as a child is fulfilling an emotional need for the parent, that cannot occur. The greater the emotional maturity of the parent, the more the child's development will be based on reality. For the child to develop adequately, the parents have the task and responsibility of functioning in ways that permit that individuality and emotional maturity to emerge.

Bowen further contends that parents typically function in ways that result in their children achieving about the same degree of emotional separation from them that they themselves achieved from their parents. The ability to develop emotionally is also tied to the characteristics of a person's relationship with parents, siblings, and other important relatives. Depending on the particular relationship each child has with the parents, one child may achieve a little more emotional separation from the parents than another child in the same family.

In families with a high level of emotional maturity, a child is permitted to grow, to think, to feel, and to act responsibly for him- or herself. This allows the child to develop individuality and achieve emotional separation from the parents. Such a child views self, parents, siblings, and others as distinct and separate individuals. The child's self-image is not formed in reaction to the anxieties and emotional neediness of others. The child can develop a consistent system of beliefs, values, and convictions. In essence, the child grows to be a part of the family, yet has the ability to emotionally separate from it.

Conversely, in families with a low level of emotional maturity, a child is not permitted to grow, to think, to feel, and to act for him- or herself. The child learns to function in reaction to others with behavior based more on emotional reactiveness than thinking. As an adult, having achieved very little emotional separation from the family, such a child continues to have dependent relationships . Such adults often still need to gain their parents' approval; they are not emotionally separated.

DETACHMENT VERSUS DISENGAGEMENT

Nearly everyone has some unresolved emotional attachment to the previous generation. However, the lower the emotional maturity, the greater the unresolved dependency in the individual's own generation, which is ultimately passed on to the next generation. A family with high dependency needs becomes enmeshed. When enmeshment exists, appropriate personal boundaries are not present. The enmeshed family has an intense sense of loyalty and closeness that minimizes disagreement among its members. Incest is more likely to occur within extremely enmeshed families..

Disengagement involves family members that have either physically and/or emotionally disassociated from the family. However, even though the members have disengaged and perhaps physically separated from the family, the conflict among the parties has not been resolved. Disengagement is simply an emotional cutoff. It is actually a symptom of enmeshment with the family of origin, because it is a means of avoiding conflict resolution. Disengaged individuals may yearn for emotional closeness to their parents, but run from it because the unresolved conflicts are too painful for them to deal with. According to Bowen, denying the importance of one's family and building an exaggerated façade of independence from the family are two sure signs of emotional cutoff and a lack of conflict resolution.

Detachment, in contrast, is a state of emotional neutrality. It requires the ability to see both sides of a relationship process between two others and make a choice to not take sides or become emotionally involved. A person's observing and thinking about what might be occurring between others is not clouded with preconceptions about what should be best for others or the misperception that he or she can help solve the problem. Any conflict that may have arisen in the past has been successfully resolved.

THE MULTIGENERATIONAL TRANSMISSION PROCESS

Projection is one of the ego-defense mechanisms of self-deception: The person assigns his or her own unacceptable thoughts and impulses to another person. In other words, it is always the *other* person's fault—the other person who initiates the behavior or behaves to cause the inappropriate action of the first person.

Bowen (Kerr & Bowen, 1988) defines projection as being part of multigenerational transmission. Multigenerational transmission is the process by which the generations pass down levels of functioning, strengths and weaknesses, and family patterns to the next generation.

Although specific behaviors may be altered from one generation to another, the basic patterns of emotional functioning and relating to others remain. Bowen describes the family projection process as the transmission of parental emotional undifferentiation, anxieties, and immaturities to a child.

The most basic component of the transmission process is the deep emotional attachment between mother and child. The more intense the unresolved symbiotic attachment, the more a child's development will be influenced by the needs and fears of his or her family. If emotional separation between a mother and a child has not been achieved, the child's image of the mother is affected by his or her own emotional needs and fears. A well-entrenched symbiotic relationship can be seen as a *mutual* projection process.

Mutual projection generally operates within the father-mother-child triangle, where it centers around the mother–child relationship. The mother usually puts the most time and energy into the children and makes the greatest emotional investment in them. The projection process begins with the mother's anxiety about the child and her concerns about her ability as a responsible parent. The child responds anxiously to the mother's anxiety, which, in turn, the mother mistakes for a problem in the child and addresses it with increased attention and overprotection. Thus, a cycle of reciprocating anxiety is set up between mother and child. The mother, in her anxiety, continues to infantilize the child, who in turn becomes increasingly more demanding and impaired. The father, pulled in by the mother–child emotionality, becomes sensitive to the mother's anxiety. To calm and reassure her, he plays a supporting role to her in dealing with the child. This completes the triangle.

Generally, parents tend to raise children to be at the same level of emotional maturity as themselves, or lower. The more intense a triangle, the more likely a child is to end up on a lower maturity level than the parents and to mate with someone of equal (low) maturity. However, a child who grows up outside this parental projection process can reach a higher level of maturity than that of the parents and select a mate of equal (higher) maturity. To alter these less functional patterns, the individual must decide to change personally and to develop neutrality about people and situations that produce emotional effects. Looking closely at the family generational relationship can reveal past patterns and provide a clue as to what is happening today. It also helps predict what is likely to occur in future generations.

Steinglass (1987) has described a systems view of alcoholism as it relates to the generational transmission process. He sees alcoholism as a continuous process occurring in family development. The family with an alcoholic member struggles with the issue of whether or not to accommodate to the alcoholism of one member and whether to include it as part of their family identity.

The family identity involves the members' attitudes and beliefs that define the family. It also incorporates their beliefs and attitudes about alcohol or chemical use. As the children form families of their own, they may organize their new families around the identity formulated by their families of origin, or may accept only part of their families' identity. Or they may have become so repelled by their childhood experience, as in an alcoholic family, that they exclude it entirely from their new family identity.

EXERCISES

1. Reflect on families you have known that have contained a symbiotic relationship. Describe that relationship.
2. Considering the chemically dependent family, describe an example of a triangle involving each of the following changes:
   a. stabilizing an unstable twosome by the addition of a third person
   b. stabilizing an unstable twosome by the removal of a third person
   c. destabilizing a stable twosome by the addition of a third person
   d. destabilizing a stable twosome by the removal of a third person
3. Within a chemically dependent family, describe a scenario in which a person shows that he or she has emotionally detached from the family.
4. Describe a scenario in which a person shows that he or she is disengaged from the family.

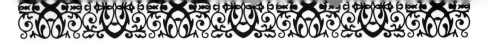

Chapter Six

Family Organizational Structure and Development

The basic family unit is a structure of people who live together and share daily life. Within that unit, and aside from all the challenges external to the family, members are challenged to balance their basic needs for belonging as an integral part of the family with that of striving for individuality. Typically, within each family unit, individuals struggle to be a part of the group and yet separate, to be alike and yet different, to be protected and yet free, to have support from the family and yet be independent.

Each newly formed family needs to clearly define itself as a separate and distinct unit, and not merely an extension of the respective families of origin. According to Steinglass (1987), fundamental developmental issues must be resolved during a family's formation. Initially, the members must define their internal and external boundaries, to determine family membership and its extent to which others are included. Further, they must choose a limited number of major developmental themes to which the family will be committed. Finally, they must develop a set of shared values and beliefs, not only about what kind of family they are, but how they are to function in society in general.

Moreover, each member often has a different perception of how his or her needs are to be fulfilled. This is a natural process in any family development. If a family system is to operate efficiently and effectively, each family member must have some assurance of his or her own worth and importance in the unit. Also, the rules under which the family functions must support each member's personal self-worth, and communication must be honest and open.

Steinglass characterizes the family's organization as involving both relationships among individual members and the family's collective patterned relationships. The stability of the family system depends on the consistency of its organizational characteristics. Consistency is achieved through the interplay of the family's organization, its internal regulation, and controlled growth.

ORGANIZATION

The organizational character of the family system reflects both all the individual members, and the family unit as a whole, like a jigsaw puzzle and its pieces. To understand the dynamics of a specific family, one must consider both the various elements of the system—the individual members and their respective characteristics—and how the various elements occur and come together within the system.

No single element within a system acts independently. The state and behaviors of each family member are constrained by, conditioned by, or dependent on the state and behaviors of all the other family members.

DEVELOPMENT

Like the individual, the family also goes through developmental stages, each with specific tasks or objectives that must be accomplished before moving on to the next stage. At the same time the family is maturing as a system, its individual members are developing. Therefore, not only do developmental issues and maturation levels of the family unit shape individual members, but the development of individuals also shapes the family unit. Failure to achieve objectives or master tasks within any developmental phase blocks family maturation.

Steinglass (1987) provides an outline of these family developmental or systemic maturation phases for the normative family. He identifies the tasks necessary to be accomplished in each phase as follows.

Early Phase: Establishing Boundaries and Identity Formation

The primary goal of the early phase is to form the family's identity. Usually the most dynamic and exciting phase for the family, it is a time of intensity, rapid change, and starting off fresh. Family members usually begin it with a sense of optimism about the future and of being able to tackle whatever comes along. During this period the family must work to establish the system boundaries and define shared rules and belief systems as a freestanding system. The basic rules for family functioning encompass such areas as distribution of tasks, allocation of personal and physical space, sexual behavior, and external friendships.

Boundaries
Each family has the responsibility to negotiate and formulate the nature of its internal and external boundaries. Boundaries are invisible barriers that surround the family system, subsystems, and individual members. Internal boundaries regulate how much contact each person has with others and protect the separateness and autonomy of the family and its individual members. They also determine the internal structure of the family. External boundaries separate the family from outsiders and define where the natural borders of the family end: who

belongs and who does not belong to the family, including extended family.

The family's established boundaries can be permeable, rigid, or diffuse. There can also be some combination of boundary types among various members, depending on the different relationships.

Permeable boundaries are clear and direct, but flexible. Family members can communicate effectively, mutually respect one another, and are considerate of each other's needs for space and privacy. Children can grow and develop emotional maturity.

Rigid boundaries are overly restrictive and inflexible. They do not provide support for one another nor allow members to move independently within the system. Family members cannot develop a solid sense of belonging. They also permit little contact with people outside the system.

Diffuse boundaries offer a high degree of mutual support, but at the expense of independence and autonomy for members. Family members tend to speak for one another, dictate to and control each other, and encroach on each other's rights and privacy. Family rules and discipline are inconsistent and, at times, too permissive. When boundaries are extremely diffuse, the members are enmeshed. The members of enmeshed families are so intertwined that they have little if any opportunity for personal growth or individuality.

Inadequate family boundaries result in boundary violations among members. Individual members never acquire a clear sense of boundary definition, and cannot define their personal emotional, physical, and relational boundaries. Emotional boundaries determine how a person is treated emotionally, and the depth of intimate expression shared with others. Behavior that violates emotional boundaries may involve sexual harassment, sexual comments and innuendos, personal questioning, sarcastic or derogatory comments, and attempts to control how members believe or feel. Physical or sexual boundaries define safe and appropriate behavior. Behavior that violates physical boundaries are incest, rape, inappropriate touching, or any physical contact that is inappropriate for the relationship. Relational boundaries establish the limits of interaction with another person, how intimate or how casual the relationship will be.

Boundaries can also be violated by distancing, or what Bradshaw (1988) refers to as "abandonment." This type of violation occurs when the amount of closeness expected as part of a relationship is not there. A distance violation occurs when a child does not receive enough attention from the parents or is subjected to broken promises. Other distancing violations include a husband refusing to discuss important matters with his wife, partners refusing to speak to each other for any period of time, or a child or a partner being deprived of appropriate touch.

Family Identity

Individual identity is one's sense of self, an awareness of who one is and, at the same time, what one shares with others. And just as individuals must develop an ego-identity, so must the family. Steinglass (1987) describes family identity as "the family's subjective sense of its own continuity over time, its present situation, and its character. As such, family identity is an underlying cognitive structure, a set of fundamental beliefs, attitudes, and attributions the family shares about itself" (p. 58).

However, Steinglass views family identity as encompassing more than the family members. Family identity has as its foundation a shared system of beliefs. This shared belief system involves the family members' assumptions about their roles, relationships, and values. Their assumptions determine how they interact with each other and with other groups. Essential characteristics of this shared belief system are the family paradigm, family themes, and family rules.

The family *paradigm* is the family's shared view of its environment, and shapes family behavior. This view is based on how the members respond to one another and how their response influences the response of others. The paradigm is a model by which a family operates in its patterned responses and interactions with each other. For example, considering oneself to be a Southerner would be to interact in a manner considered characteristic of the South.

Family *themes* are those patterns of feelings, motives, fantasies, and understandings that typify the family's view of reality and how it is organized as a unit. They are the constructed realities to which the family unit adheres and becomes the family's concept of who it is and how they portray it. Themes are very narrow definitions of the family as a whole unit and as individuals, and are needed by the family to keep its precarious balance. They essentially make the statement "We are this way and can't help it and the same is true for others; we cannot relate in any other way than our way." These are sometimes referred to as family myths. A family theme might be, for example, "We, the Baskervilles, always make a good impression."

Family *rules* link the parts of a family system to accomplish a common purpose. The rules determine how family members relate to one another and to outsiders. Rules generally support and preserve the family themes. For example, the following rules might support the example theme just given:

"We never talk to others about our problems."
"We never let anyone see us cry."
"We never show our anger."

The rules can be quite explicit and can establish

- who may talk to whom and about what
- when and how a family member may leave the family to relate to others, or to be alone
- when and how a member may differ from or resemble another
- how one may be unique, and how, when, and where one may exhibit that uniqueness
- what, when, and how one may comment on what one sees, feels, and thinks
- how one may show feelings such as love, hurt, and anger, and how one may receive those feelings from another
- how and when one may let needs and wants be known to another and respond to the needs and wants of others
- how one may feel and express sexuality
- how one may gain self-esteem and how much one may have
- how one may grow and change in another's presence and how one may be a man or a woman and a human being

John Bradshaw (1988) posits that the most important family rules are fundamental beliefs about raising children. What parents believe about human life and fulfillment regulates how they raise their children. These beliefs include ingrained attitudes such as what it means to be a woman or a man, expectations placed on others, and how children are to behave. Family rules are formulated to support those beliefs. The resulting parenting style, in turn, forms the child's core beliefs about what it means to be a human being and about him- or herself. To allow mature development, family rules must be flexible, particularly with regard to ordinary developmental changes. As children grow and mature, they must be allowed more freedom, methods of discipline must be modified, and the relationship between parent and child must change.

Bradshaw notes that rules about raising children are generally considered the most sacred of all rules and are often reinforced by religious teaching and school systems. Within a functional family, children are allowed to question the validity of specific rules and to request compromise, and parents feel free to consider or make compromise. Within a dysfunctional family, questioning rules is considered an act of disobedience and a dishonor to the parents. Here lie denial and no-talk rules, such as "Children speak only when spoken to; children obey all adults without question; children are seen and not heard." Bradshaw declares that these kinds of rules are abusive and shaming to a child because they destroy any sense of inner identity. As an adult, "the child within" continues to obey such rules and pass them down to the next generation.

Steinglass (1987) considers that family identity "incorporates certain beliefs about family members—who belongs and who does not, both now and in the past." Although family connectedness or membership may not be sensed at a conscious level, most families tend to preserve their identity, at least to some degree, from one generation to the next.

Most partners in a couple are part of and influenced by the family identities of both their families of origin in attempting to establish an identity of the newly formed family. At times, particularly during major developmental transitions, considerable conflict may arise because each partner wants to impose his or her family-of-origin values, rules, and beliefs on the newly created family. For instance, when a family is establishing its manner of disciplining the children, conflict may arise depending on how discipline was handled in the families of origin.

According to Steinglass, at each generational transition a family faces three fundamentally different choices with regard to its identity: to continue as is into the next generation, to blend aspects of both families of origin, or to assume a new family identity. If the family believes that alcoholism is a central organizing principle for family life, then the continuance of this core identity will heavily determine whether or not alcoholism is transmitted to another generation. In other words, if a family has accommodated to the alcoholism by how it functions day by day, the activities conducted to sustain the drinking will likely be continued to the next generation. For example, perhaps the only time the family rallies together is when the alcoholic is intoxicated.

If the family's core identity is maintained at each generational transition level, the family will take on what Steinglass terms "dynastic qualities." Such qualities are the family's ability to establish powerful shared beliefs and traditions that demand full adherence by all members across multiple generations. In a family dynasty, individual identity is based on membership in the family, which demands the loyalty of all members. If family dynasty is built around economic or political power, for example, one might be a Kennedy, a Roosevelt, or a Ford. Family members tend to feel their life course must follow the dictates of that dynastic identity.

A family dynasty can also be built around alcoholism or addiction. When it survives across multiple generations, it may produce an alcoholic dynastic identity. The demands of that identity may influence members' beliefs, attitudes, and behavioral expectations toward alcoholism or addiction. For example, if a family believes that manhood is exemplified by heavy consumption of alcohol and that drinking is a normal part of life, that belief can be carried into successive generations, so alcoholism can be expected.

Family Growth

The general purpose of the family unit is to create an environment or a framework within which mature, fully functioning individuals can develop. However, the extent to which family members are able to grow and develop emotionally depends on how well the individuals in the family are contributing to and participating in the family process. In other words, depending on the individuals' emotional maturity, the family unit is either in a "growth" or an "arrested" framework. As with individuals, the family has basic needs of survival, belonging, esteem, and individuality that must be met.

Growth framework To the degree that a family is operating in a framework that fosters growth, it can achieve these basic needs and become more fully functioning as a unit. The degree of family differentiation is directly related to the emotional maturity and individuality achieved by its separate members. Likewise, individual maturity of the members is directly related to that of the family unit. In other words, individuals must maintain their separate identities while simultaneously maintaining unity with the other family members.

For a family to be in a *growth framework*, certain basic concepts need to exist. Family members must be able to accept individual differences. They must realize the fact that at times tension will be generated in their attempt to balance the needs of the core group with those of individuals. In decision making, the family interaction must take into consideration the presenting circumstances and individual feelings. Members must be able to maintain flexible behavior and attitude by making allowances and compromises based on both family and individual needs. Family members must have a sense of availability, commitment, and unconditional love to and from each other. When conflict arises, each family member must try to become aware of and take responsibility for personal feelings and thoughts. They must be able to feel free to share or not share these feelings and thoughts as appropriate to the situation.

In a growth-enhanced or functional family, the rules allow for individual separation and emotional maturity. One member may talk to another about experienced reactions, observations, thoughts, or feelings, or choose not to do so, but the reason is not to protect or enhance self-esteem. Members value self and others, judging one another's perceptions is not an issue, and ulterior motives do not govern statements or actions. Responses of others to what one member says are heard as additional information and do not lessen the value of self or the people who offer such responses. One can listen and hear feelings as expressed by others, and when hearing conflicting messages, is free to confront or comment on them. The person can feel opposite reactions toward the same person.

Family members are comfortable with negative feedback and are able to benefit from constructive input. Relationships with members of the previous generation are nonintrusive so that a healthy separation of the generations is maintained. Members of the family have equality and are free to periodically select a specific role within the family as circumstances may dictate. For instance, an older daughter may take over care of younger siblings while the mother is in the hospital but relinquishes the role when the mother has recuperated. Family members are free to express their individual differences. Role structure, positioning, and expectations can be negotiated. Members are available to each other as the need arises. The family protects each individual's aloneness, belongingness, and uniqueness. Healthy families look for ways to enlarge on their experiences and can continue growing despite whatever crises or problems are encountered.

In a healthy family, going in and out of the family has to do with individual and family needs as they occur, such as learning to establish one's own home but returning to help out in emergency situations. Behavior is not used to send indirect messages, nor is it interpreted in a stereotyped way. Each member is free to develop uniqueness as a human being, and whether that will be similar to or different from another is not relevant. Everyone in the family can be aware of needs and wants without judgment. Members can express needs without fear of rejection, and what needs and wants are met are commensurate with the present context and the choices of others.

Sexuality consists of those individual characteristics that define personal gender identity. It is an important part of life. In a healthy family, the expression of sexuality is acceptable and need not be hidden or expressed by a rigid rule, but may be expressed by choice, as is appropriate to the context of what is occurring.

Self-esteem is not diminished by attack or blame; it is a basic ingredient of a healthy family. When one member is experiencing situational low self-esteem, others attempt to support positively that person's innate worth as a person. Movement toward further realization of each individual's potential is celebrated. Retreat for introspection is also honored by the family. Members follow their own inner guides toward achieving autonomy, and family members support one another in the effort to do so.

Arrested framework If a family is in an arrested framework, its members develop maladaptive or ineffective communication styles. Family members tend to project their problems onto each other. One or more individuals strive to maintain a rigid position in the family, and members subscribe to family role expectations rather than seeking self-development and self-identity. Within this framework, individual growth is limited.

Within a dysfunctional family, the rules generally do not allow individual separation and individuation. Members are not allowed to ask questions, particularly in sensitive areas. Expression of what one really thinks and feels is restricted; or else all things seen or felt are expected to become family property. Members may not express pain and anger verbally. Either members must be careful about how much caring is expressed, so as not to embarrass anyone, or must continually express love feelings, whether they're felt or not, to make certain of not offending anyone. Communication is faulty and indirect. For example, if the child wants the father to know something, the child tells the mother, who tells the father.

If someone is alone or prefers to be with others, that person is suspected of not caring about family members or of being angry. Differences among family members are completely obscured. If someone responds to the needs of others, the label "strong" is assigned to that person; the other will wear the label "weak." Individuals either do not say what they want for themselves, expecting others to know, or always express every need or want and demand fulfillment regardless of the circumstances.

Sexuality is either dismissed by the arrested family or, conversely, is always the major facet of one's being, and inappropriately expressed. Self-esteem depends on how well one follows the family rules. Children may not surpass their parents in self-esteem. Personal change is controlled so that people remain as similar as possible to how they have been in the past. The family has rigid standards, expressed in formulas such as "Men always . . . Women always . . ."

The outcome of the early phase is the gradual emergence of a family identity that subsequently serves as one of the major regulatory principles for the family's life.

Middle Phase: Commitment and Stability

Steinglass places the primary emphasis of the middle phase on maintaining a stable and predictable family environment. It is the longest phase, and can be a period of tremendous richness, accomplishment, and exciting new adventures for the family. The central themes of family life established in the early phase are now in place. This period now becomes a time of orderly consolidation and commitment to a limited number of central organization themes. The family has established a set of stable and consistent rules regarding role behavior and relationships. This phase is dominated by regulatory rather than growth forces.

Internal Regulation

A family's stability is constantly being challenged. There are, for instance, economic conditions, political decisions, and the demands of society at large over which the family has no control and that exert external challenges. Internally the family confronts the personal agendas, psychological needs, and physical demands of individual family members. In the presence of these challenges, the family system requires some process by which it can maintain some stability. In addition, family behavior is generally patterned and predictable. For a family to regulate its life and remain stable, it needs some mechanisms to organize structure and determine the rules that control responsive or patterned behavior.

Steinglass concludes that regulatory processes allow the family to maintain or to reestablish stability after some event or circumstance that has disrupted homeostasis. These mechanisms include the family's daily routines, ritualistic behavior, and the way it handles short-term problem solving. Daily routines and family rituals can also be affected by other factors, such as making allowances for a member's work schedule. However, when these patterned behaviors focus on adapting to the chemically dependent's use and behavior, the chemical dependency has affected the family's internal regulation.

Steinglass (1987), in identifying essential features of the homeostatic model of regulation, compares it to a thermostat. A family can only function optimally within a limited range. Therefore, the family must keep its internal environment within that range. Verbal or nonverbal cues among family members operate on a feedback loop to serve as sensory devices, continually monitoring the parameters within which a family can function. An attempt to function outside those parameters disrupts the homeostatic regulation. Say, for instance, a family's limited range extends between 45 and 80 degrees on the "thermostat." Changes in behavior, responses, or member interaction so great that the family functioning may become chaotic, indicate that the temperature has fallen below 45 or exceeds 80 degrees.

An emotionally mature family's optimal functioning range is fairly expansive. It can also generally recognize an imbalance, can adequately assess the situation, and make allowances and adjustments to return to optimal functioning. Less emotionally mature families have a narrower range of optimal functioning. Unfortunately, some families simply cannot sense when they've moved outside their acceptable range so that the necessary adjustment can be made. Other families can sense that something is wrong, but they respond with inappropriate or ineffective behaviors.

Steinglass further denotes three basic categories of observable family behavior that helps identify underlying family regulatory processes or indicates how the family functions. These groups of behavior are the family's daily routines, rituals, and method of short-term problem solving.

Daily routines Behaviors that provide the structure within which the family lives on a daily basis are daily routines. They consist of regulated activities such as meals, the sleep/wake cycle, housekeeping duties, shopping, and the use of space in the home.

Family rituals Family activities that are established and trans-mitted from one generation to the next are family rituals. Types of behaviors that become ritualized for families are

> family celebrations such as religious and secular holidays, and rites of passage
> less culture-specific family traditions that involve recurrent be-haviors that are considered special and meaningful to the family, such as birthdays, family vacations, and family reunions
> patterned routines, such as bedtime, dinnertime, or leisure activities

Families differ in how much variance they can tolerate in their rituals. Rigid families tolerate very few if any deviations in rituals. Other families allow modification or revision of rituals by certain family members for what seem to be valid reasons. Still other families are even more flexible toward ritual life and let children gain power in the family as they mature. In flexible families, the rituals have value but variations are allowed and even encouraged.

Short-term problem solving Over time, a family develops a style of problem solving. The style may be proactive or reactive, calm or intense, cohesive or divisive. The degree to which family members have acquired effective and appropriate problem-solving skills determines their ability to resolve problems and restabilize. Healthy families consider both the benefits and consequences, both short and long term, that may result from their choices. Unhealthy families tend to make spur-of-the-moment decisions without considering possible consequences or other alterna-tives. This style keeps them continually facing crises.

Controlled Growth

Controlled growth involves family growth, change, development, and a tendency to become organizationally more complex over time. Such controls involve the deeper regulatory structures of the family. These regulatory principles operate within the family's boundaries and govern how guidelines or rules are established for the family's patterned behavior. They are located deep within the core of the family and function rather like a family command center.

The outcome of the middle phase is the emergence of a set of repetitive and highly structured behavioral programs for organizing the family's daily routines, special events, and strategies for solving problems of daily living. Families unable to make these shifts remain fixated at the early phase of development.

Late Phase: Clarification and Legacy

During the late phase, the family's focus shifts from the present to the future. Children are leaving home and perhaps starting families of their own. Parents may be planning for retirement. It is a time of restabilization and reorganization. Instead of initiating family themes and boundaries, members are placed in the position of defending them, particularly to the grown children and their mates. Identity issues have likely become more implicit than explicit, and the family has experienced a lot of changes since its initial formation. Being challenged by new members with new ideas begins to strain the ability of the family regulatory behaviors to maintain stability. However, the healthy family usually can restabilize and incorporate the new members and new ideas with minimal disruption.

EXERCISES

1. Describe and discuss an example of a situation that may occur in families (a) with permeable boundaries, (b) with rigid boundaries, and (c) diffuse boundaries. How might each situation be handled by the family?
2. Identify four or five typical family themes and their supporting rules.
3. Describe a critical or traumatic situation that might occur in a family, and how a well-differentiated family might go about restabilizing or regaining homeostasis after such a crisis.

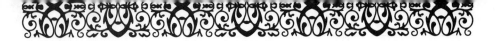

Chapter Seven

Chemical Dependency's Disruption of Organization

Dr. Steinglass (1987) has analyzed the characteristics of "the alcoholic family" within Bowen's family systems theory. He concludes that even if only one member is the identified alcoholic, it is possible for the entire family to "have alcoholism." This phenomenon exists when alcohol-related behavior has been so deeply incorporated into family functioning that it plays a crucial role in the family's daily life. Because almost any significant mental or physical illness can have a similar impact on a family system, this conclusion can reasonably be extended to include dependency on any drug.

In "the alcoholic family," or chemically dependent family, behavior related to alcohol or drug use plays a major role in the family system. Family homeostasis and growth have become organized around and distorted by chemical dependency. Family development has become distorted by incorporating an alcohol/drug life history. However, in some families chemical dependency is not incorporated into the family's organizational system. According to Steinglass, even though the family has somewhat accommodated to the chemical dependency, it would not necessarily be considered a "chemically dependent family."

The presence of chemical dependency can severely affect the family's regulatory processes. The chemically dependent family typically has established environmental limits that are too inappropriately narrow— or inappropriately wide—to activate corrective homeostatic mechanisms. The characteristic rigidity of the family's regulatory mechanisms might result in a tendency for the members to set their "internal thermostats" for an inappropriately narrow range. Using the thermostat metaphor, for instance, the family's optimal range of functioning might be only 60 to 75 degrees, rather than 45 to 90 degrees. Therefore, the slightest change in the environmental "temperature," forcing them outside this limited range, can be extremely distressing to the family. For instance, a family might adapt to a member's short-term illness at home but fall apart under the circumstance of a member being hospitalized. The family members may then react in chaotic and explosive ways.

As previously indicated, any family regularly confronts challenges, not only normal developmental issues, but also unplanned emer- gencies, influences, or circumstances. Confronting and resolving these challenges provides the family and its members with opportunities to grow and mature. However, the chemically dependent family generally emphasizes the short-term stability of family life, setting aside other important issues that are necessary for family growth confronting the family. The family interprets any challenge to short-term stability primarily as a threat to its structure. Family members are likely to overreact to any developmental or external challenge they confront rather than taking a proactive approach to the challenge. In doing so, they ignore the possibilities for growth normally inherent in these challenges.

INTERNAL REGULATION

Steinglass believes that the family's established regulatory mechanisms maintain stability, order, and control of systems functioning. These mechanisms regulate overall patterns of family behavior. Such behavior patterns are differentially receptive to chronic addiction. That is, some family styles are not at all compatible with its existence; it continues to create dissonance or tension in the family. Other family styles can be conducive to the existence of chemical dependency; it has been so accepted as a fact of life that the members' lives are built around it and may become dependent on it. As noted, the regulatory mechanisms can themselves be taken over by chemical dependency and related behavior. In other words, the regulatory behaviors actually alter so as to make them more compatible with chemical dependency. For example, a mother going to work to adequately support the family because the father has lost his job can alter the family's schedule for meals or other activities. Under these circumstances, the dependency itself contributes to the family's unity and stability.

According to Steinglass, once chemical dependency becomes integrated into the family's organizational structure, it is maintained by the family's regulatory behaviors rather than being contained or eliminated from the family's life. For instance, family short-term problem-solving strategies can actually come to rely on alcohol- or drug-related behavior to bring an issue to surface. For example, poor family financial management might never be discussed until brought up in a heated dispute related to the alcohol/drug behavior.

In chemically dependent families, regulated activities are often vague and become even more inconsistent with progression of the dependency. A family's level of functioning can be ascertained from the regulatory process or from the family's patterned behavior. Steinglass identifies chemical dependency's impact on the family's daily routines, rituals, and its manner of short-term problem solving, as follows.

Daily Routines

The patterns of the family's daily routines reflect and reinforce the underlying regulatory principles related to chemical dependency. Therefore, looking at how and to what extent the family patterns have changed over time to be compatible with chemical dependency, can show how daily functioning has been affected. These alterations can be related to any day-to-day functions that are a normal part of life. They include such activities as mealtimes, bedtimes, and chore scheduling. One woman complained to me that she wasn't getting enough sleep because she had to sit up and wait for her intoxicated husband to wake up, because he had fallen asleep in a chair. When I asked why, she replied, "Well, his head drops over, and he might break his neck." Her daily routine was affected by his behavior.

Family Rituals

The extent to which family rituals are protected or not protected from involvement with the dependency-related behavior also indicates the family's functioning. Chemical dependency easily disrupts family rituals. For example, the family might move the time for opening gifts from Christmas Eve to Christmas morning because the chemically dependent member begins his or her celebration after work. Or the family might decline the traditional Thanksgiving dinner at grandmother's house because of the dependent's "traditional" intoxication. As the disease progresses, the more rituals will likely be disrupted, to ensure that the chemically dependent member can continue to be included in these events. The family often must work hard at preserving rituals to keep them from being disrupted or taken over by the issues related to chemical dependency.

Short-Term Problem Solving

All families face day-to-day challenges. However, in the chemically dependent family the problems are more likely to create tension and anxiety rather than to evoke an attempt at effective resolution. In the chemically dependent family, problems often seem to be a necessary element of the family members relating to one another. The only time family members show some cohesiveness is when they face a crisis. Some such families invent problems that don't actually exist. In the chemically dependent family, blaming others for problems tends to become the normal way to avoid resolution. Problems are often easily activated, and responses to them disproportionately overreactive in relation to the magnitude of the problem. Some behavior or problems, of course, only occur or are only activated during periods of active drug use. For example, they may attempt to discuss the issue of who manages the bank account because one party considers it to be mismanaged by the other. When specific problems arise only under these circumstances, the drug use has itself become a regulating factor for the family.

Steinglass concludes that chemically dependent families tend to misinterpret and mismanage normative developmental changes, assuming that they are unacceptable threats to their overall homeostasis. Because the chemically dependent family and its behavior are organized around maintaining short-term stability, family members tend to overreact to developmental issues. Families in which chemical dependency exists have highly complex behavioral systems. Although they may seem to have remarkable stability, they increasingly achieve stability at the expense of resiliency and adaptability. When developmental or environmental demands finally exceed the family's ability to maintain balance, the family usually considers the situation catastrophic. However, some chemically dependent families show remarkable tolerance for stress for long periods, with only intermittent adaptive behavioral reactiveness.

Steinglass acknowledges that families can be affected differently by chemical dependency. Chemical dependency in some families may be associated with a family's coping style centered around an attempt to isolate the chemically dependent individual. These attempts can be intended to keep the family's secret from outsiders or to preserve the dependent's reputation. The isolation may also be manifested by making excuses or covering up for inappropriate behavior to both outsiders and family members. The purpose, either intentionally or unintentionally, is to protect other family members from possible consequences of the intoxicated behavior. Isolation also lets the family emphasize its perceived values of self-reliance, seeking to convey the message that it needs nothing, from no one. Isolation also conveys the family's lowered expectations of what is acceptable for family functioning.

In other families, the drug-related behavior may go virtually unnoticed or be ignored by other family members. Such families have established a well-developed system of denial. The situation is marked by the premise "If you don't see it, it isn't there" or "If it is ignored, it will go away."

Still other families view chemical dependency as inevitable, as a predetermined built-in feature of life closely linked to the family's cultural or ethnic values. This attitude is particularly derived through the generational transmission process when addiction has been present for a number of generations. Here a tremendous amount of accommodation has been made to the chemical dependency.

And, finally, there are always those families that may be fully aware of the dreadful consequences chemical dependency is imposing on their lives, but are still helpless to develop an effective strategy for coping with it. Their helplessness may be the result of ignorance that something might be done to intervene, or they may not be willing to risk a family breakup, or may simply fear that the chemically dependent will become violent when confronted. Instead of attempting an effective solution, the family generates a chaotic reactiveness to each confrontation, in an attempt to restabilize.

IMPACT ON FAMILY DEVELOPMENTAL STAGES

Steinglass (1987) further denotes the manner in which chemical dependency can disrupt or retard the family's developmental process.

Early Phase

The developmental objectives in the early phase are to establish family internal and external boundaries and form family identity. In families where chemical dependency exists, these tasks are essentially the same as for any family. The basic difference is that whenever chemical dependency surfaces, the family faces a crucial decision: whether to challenge the associated behavior or accommodate to it.

According to Steinglass, with the emergence of chemical dependency, very important concerns become relevant to the early-phase family. First, chemical dependency can preempt development. That is, it proves so powerful and compelling a force in family life that all other issues tend to be ignored. The rules governing interpersonal relationships within the family begin to revolve around rules for interpreting and managing drug-affected behavior. For instance, they might be related to when it's unsafe to talk to Dad in association with his chemical use, or being unable to invite friends over because they might see the dependent at his or her worst. Also, delineation of external boundaries often centers around who is to be let in on the addiction issue and how the information is to be shared with others. It may be okay to let Uncle Ben know, but don't say anything to Grandmother.

Furthermore, individuals are powerfully influenced by their families of origin. A family's shared perception of chemical dependency as transmitted from one generation to another will dictate very different response patterns for the newly formed family. Depending on which side of the issue it has taken, the family's shared perception can determine whether or not it will be tolerated. Families still have many options available to them in this phase of development as they respond to drug-affected behavior, particularly if chemical use has not yet developed into chronic dependency.

Another crucial issue mentioned by Steinglass arises at this phase of family development. This involves deciding which aspects of the respective families of origin will be incorporated into the new family. The family also must decide on how deliberately it will preserve those aspects. These heritage identities may, for example, revolve around careers, educational levels, or family size. If the family heritage includes chemical dependency, the family may decide to continue that heritage even though the use at this stage is not problematic. Or the family may extend an active use pattern along the lines already defined by a chemically dependent parent. They may also develop a new nondependency identity that excludes alcohol or drug use. Finally, the family may just leave the issue unresolved.

Chemical dependency affects family identity formation in two instances. The first instance is when the family enters the early phase with an already established problem of dependency. The other instance is when chemical dependency arises while the family is working out its identity issues. In either case, the challenge to the family is whether or not to adjust or to accommodate to chemical dependency as a "fact of life" or to effectively exclude it from all important aspects of life. When a family adjusts and accommodates, chemical dependency will, over time, probably become an integral part of the family's emerging identity. In other words, the family will adopt a "chemically dependent family" identity.

Middle Phase

Committing to a set of family norms that will ensure stability is the major task for the middle phase of development. The chemically dependent family builds maintenance activities around a core of alcohol- or drug-related behaviors. The dependent person very rarely adjusts his or her use to accommodate to the family. Rather, the other family members must adapt their lives to the dependent's use and behaviors. They strike a balance between stabilizing family life and disrupting as little as possible the needs of the chemically dependent family member. Thus, chemical dependency increasingly plays a central role, not only in the family's sense of itself, but also in the very behavior used to regulate and control family life.

Under these conditions, orderly growth cannot occur, because the family emphasizes a set of rigid homeostatic mechanisms and are inflexibly committed to keeping things just as they are. This profoundly alters the customary trend toward family development. With chemical dependency playing a central role, short-term stability becomes paramount to the family system, at the expense of orderly long-term growth.

At this point in family development, because chemical dependency invades the family regulatory behaviors, behavior among family members very likely has fundamentally altered. If the members have accommodated to the alcohol or drug use instead of confronting it, the family has become developmentally more rigid. Both family and individual growth have becomes stifled. Steinglass considers that during this middle phase the seeds of generational transmission of chemical dependency are being sown.

Late Phase

Because the family's identity is fairly firmly established, the major task for the family in the late stage is that of reorganizing and stabilizing as it plans for the future. By this phase of development, chemically dependent families have developed extremely rigid boundaries and regulatory behaviors. If the family has continued on and remained intact to this stage, tremendous accommodation to the alcohol- or drug-related behavior has likely occurred. Significant developmental distortion has set in.

During this time, generational transmission of alcoholism or addiction can clearly be seen. True, there are both a biological genetic and a cultural perspective involved in the etiology of addiction. Of equal importance, however, is the transmission of personal beliefs and values regarding the use of alcohol or drugs. These particular beliefs and values are more familial than cultural or societal. The family has established a unique perspective regarding not only the use of alcohol and drugs but also how their values and behavior are related to its use. This perspective is incorporated into the "family culture" that is then transmitted to the children. This factor becomes paramount in a newly forming family in deciding whether to accept the use of alcohol or drugs or to tolerate the related behavior.

During the late phase, the family determines different options or directions in response to major developmental tasks, particularly regarding its "chemically dependent family identity." The family is now forced to make an explicit statement about chemical dependency. The nature of that statement determines which of the possible options or pathways the family will follow.

Steinglass (1987) mentions four distinct pathways or options to which alcoholic families are directed. In the following summaries, I have substituted the term "chemically dependent" for "alcoholic."

The Stable Wet Dependent Family

The first option is evidence of an accommodation of the family to the chemical dependency and its related consequences. It calls for the least amount of energy on the part of the family. For all intents and purposes, the family has taken a firm stance and has given every indication that they anticipate continued dependency despite any likely consequences. Individual family members may periodically challenge and question the wisdom of this way of life. They may threaten to leave unless change occurs, or even attempt to create a crisis intended to force an end to the use. However, these tactics do not alter the basic use-affected regulatory structure of the family. The many potential options for growth and change that might have been attempted earlier in the family's development are no longer available. The family seems to have lost not only its ability, but its will to change.

The Stable Wet or Controlled Use Nondependent Family

With the stable or controlled use option, although drinking or drug use may not stop, there is movement away from the dependency as a core developmental or family identity issue. The dependent may reduce consumption from time to time. Significantly, however, drug use is no longer the controlling factor in the family regulatory behavior. In this scenario, the family can move away from the dependent family identity without the change being necessarily accompanied by a complete cessation of use by the dependent member.

The Stable Dry Dependent Family

Within the third framework the family has successfully negotiated or coerced a conversion to nonuse by the dependent, but there is no movement away from the dependent family identity. In other words, drug(s) continues to play a central role in family life even though the dependent member is no longer actively using. In this scenario, the only thing that has changed is that the dependent has stopped using. Behavior patterns that have been established around the dependent continue to dominate family life. Family members, as well as the dependent, may still be preoccupied with the drug(s) and its related concerns.

The Stable Dry Nondependent Family

The fourth option presumes not only that has the drug use stopped, but also that the family has given up its preoccupation with drugs and drug-related issues. Some families make no particular commitment to reorganize the family; they just no longer focus on drug-related behavior and issues. Other families are more proactive in making significant changes individually and as a family unit. This stage, for them, does not merely resolve issues related to the dependency, but also involves a major family reorganization and transformation of individual members.

EXERCISES

1. Describe two or three ways in which family rituals might be disrupted by chemical dependency, in addition to the examples given in this chapter.
2. Describe two examples of problems normally encountered by a family, and show how they may be dealt with in a chemically dependent family.
3. Describe two ways in which family rituals can be disrupted by chemical dependency, and list steps the affected families might take to preserve their rituals.
4. Give two examples of ways in which family homeostasis and growth have been distorted by or organized around the presence of chemical dependency.
5. How might a family's short-term problem-solving strategies come to rely on alcohol- or drug-related behavior?
6. Describe one example each of a situation in which a new family
   a. decides to continue an alcoholic heritage
   b. extends an active drinking pattern
   c. develops a new nonalcoholic identity
   d. leaves the issue unresolved
7. Outline two situations or events that might be considered a threat to the family's structure where chemical dependency exists.
8. What strategies might the chemically dependent family use to protect family members from possible consequences of intoxicated behavior?

Chapter Eight

Critical Issues in Chemically Dependent Families

The most vulnerable members of any family are children. The impact of chemical dependency on the family's regulatory structure and interactional patterns can in themselves create adverse outcomes for developing children. Rules and disciplinary inconsistencies, the projection of blame, extreme rigidity or lack of boundary definition, lack of trust, and role confusion are all fairly typical in chemically dependent families. These conditions, of course, can and usually do become more severe with the progression of the dependency. However, even more crucial issues, such as physical and/or sexual abuse, may arise.

Although a causal relationship has not been indisputably proved, a number of studies have shown a high correlation of spousal and child abuse with alcohol or drug consumption, particularly among heavy users. What is apparent, alcohol and drugs, at the very least, serve as a disinhibiting factor in many cases of child sexual abuse and domestic violence. When sober, people can often control their expression of anger and rage or sexual fantasies. Alcohol or drugs diminish inhibition, and then the user may act out these kinds of expressions.

CHILD ABUSE

Walker, Bonner, and Kaufman (1988) found that both alcohol and drug addiction can be associated with physical abuse of children. Beasley (1987) considered that alcohol use was a factor in 38% of cases of child abuse. Other researchers have noted an even larger relationship. In New York City, Chasnoff (1988) found that alcohol and/or drug abuse was involved in 64% of all child abuse. Bays (1990) suggests that at least 675,000 children each year are seriously mistreated by an alcoholic or drug abusing caretaker. According to Bradshaw (1988), the mistreatment and abuse of their own children results from parents never being able to get their own needs met as children. The abuse is their attempt to achieve a sense of completion and to regain the power they lost to their own parents.

Bradshaw delineates the sexual abuse involved in families into four categories. Physical sexual abuse is any kind of touching in a sexual way, ranging from sexualized hugging or kissing to actual sexual intercourse. Overt sexual abuse involves voyeurism or exhibitionism. Covert sexual abuse consists of verbal expression of inappropriate sexual comments, discussions, or name calling. It also includes boundary violation, wherein children may witness their parents engaging in sexual acts, or allowing children to walk in on them in the bathroom, or seeing them nude. Emotional sexual abuse involves a parent's inappropriate bonding with a child to get his or her emotional needs met, at the expense of the child.

Bradshaw further notes the collusion that often occurs in an incestuous family. If the father is victimizing the children, the mother may collude with him. She may actively collude with him if she is aware of the sexual abuse and allows it to continue or actually participates in it. Or she may passively collude with the husband by blocking out awareness of what is occurring. In either case, the mother is guilty of failing to protect the victimized child.

Sexual or physical abuse can severely traumatize children. As adults, victims may attempt to deal with the resulting emotional pain by drug use themselves. Burnam and others (1989) found a strong relationship between women's substance abuse and previous sexual assault. A number of authors have linked an internalized sense of shame related to childhood abuse, to the dysfunctional behaviors of adult children of alcoholics.

SHAME

Shame is a clinically defined factor that is also associated with chemically dependent systems. Fossom and Mason (1986) define shame as "an inner sense of being completely diminished or insufficient as a person . . . the ongoing premise that one is fundamentally bad, inadequate, defective, unworthy, or not fully valid as a human being." Shame differs from guilt. Shame is an intensely painful feeling about one's self as a person and can seriously retard emotional growth. Guilt, in contrast, constitutes regret for an action and presents the opportunity to assert personal values, make amends, and to grow from the experience. In other words, guilt says, "I've done a bad thing," while shame says, "I am bad."

Fossom and Mason suggest that a shame-bound family operates according to rules that demand control, perfectionism, blame, and denial. Under such rules, authentic intimate relationships cannot develop. Secrets and vague personal boundaries are pervasive. Under these circumstances, family members internalize shame that is perpetuated in themselves and their relatives. This shame-bound system can arise despite the family's good intentions and love, which also may exist.

Fossom and Mason further allege that shame-bound systems can exhibit addictive, compulsive, abusive, or phobic behavior, or some combination of these behaviors. In chemically dependent families, members often go to elaborate means to keep the addiction secret from each other and from others. In addition, chemical dependency is frequently associated with physical, sexual, or emotional abuse and neglect, which is also kept secret. Secrets sustain the unhealthy balance of the system by preventing family members from changing their behavior, perpetuating the addiction and the shame of the involved members.

Kaufman (1985) proposes that shame stems from a single developmental process that takes a pathway either to a healthy self or to a shame-bound self. If a child's basic needs are not met by the parents, the child internalizes that failure as a personal failure. Consistent repetition of the shame experience is incorporated into the child's identity and further contributes to feelings of hopelessness. Under these circumstances a child is unable to develop an adequate sense of self and emotional maturity. A child's shame resulting from sexual abuse creates a skewed concept of sexuality and an inability to form meaningful mature relationships as an adult. According to Kaufman, a shame-inducing reaction in a child can be replaced by a parent with an affirming one if the parent can admit and accept responsibility for the interaction, thereby relieving the child's feeling of failure. Unfortunately, this corrective action occurs all too infrequently with chemically dependent or codependent parents.

DOMESTIC VIOLENCE

Collins and Messerschmidt (1993) suggest that alcohol abuse is involved in 60% to 70% of domestic violence cases. Gelles (1974) found that alcohol was used by 48% of the batterers studied. Sonkin and others (1985) report that over 80% of their cases involved alcohol or other drugs in the latest violent episode reported. An analysis of their intake/assessment data of 42 men they had treated revealed that 62% were under the influence of alcohol or other drugs at the last battering incident. His breakdown of a correlation between the violence and consumption revealed that 43% had been violent both while under the influence and while not under the influence, 29% had been violent only when not under the influence, and 29% had been violent only when under the influence. Of this group, 46% scored on an alcohol screening test as having an alcohol problem. They also observed that men living with alcoholic or drug-abusing women will often justify their violence against them as a way of controlling their behavior.

Although domestic violence and child abuse may present themselves in families where chemical dependency does not exist, their existence correlates highly with the use of alcohol and/or drugs. Roberts (1984) asserts that professionals working with domestic violence must first assess the alcohol/drug use of both perpetrator and victim. Particularly when abuse occurs only with alcohol/drug use, the initial focus of treatment should be stopping the chemical use and possible removal of the perpetrator from the home.

Domestic violence involving only the adult members of the family can still have a traumatic impact on the children. Parents are role models. As violent behavior is modeled, the children's interpretation of how a relationship should function becomes significantly skewed. Sonkin's analysis of the 42 batterers also revealed that 83% had received physical punishment as a child and 50% either saw their mother abused or were themselves abused. Also, 17% of this group were sexually abused as children. It cannot be assumed that violence occurs in all families where chemical dependency exists. However, because violence is prevalent in such a large percentage of chemically dependent homes, the possibility of its existence should be explored.

FAMILY SURVIVAL ROLES

The distorted regulatory structure of the chemically dependent family has an emotional impact, to some extent, on all its members. Each responds to the dependent person from his or her own perspective and individual interpretation of the family's condition and needs. In varying degrees, each member may make assumptions about his or her personal responsibility for the dependent's use and the increasing family dysfunction. This guilt, and futile attempts to make things better for the family, are likely to be associated with much internalized pain and anger. To protect themselves from further pain, family members tend to repress their true feelings. In doing so, each member develops his or her own perception of what is wrong with the family and what can be done to fulfill the family needs.

The chemical use provides an escape and a means of emotional survival for the chemically dependent person. However, other family members, to cope with the increasing dysfunction created by the dependency, may adopt various survival roles. These survival roles let the members develop a wall of defenses to cover up and protect the painful feelings they're actually experiencing and to make them "fit" within the unit. Each role fills a specific purpose in helping the family maintain homeostasis.

The growing action/reaction dilemma of the dependent and the family is self-deluding. As individual protective barriers intensify and strengthen, the entire family grows more out of touch with the reality of their emotions. As the dependent person's compulsion to use grows, so does the dysfunction increase between the dependent's erratic behavior and the family's reactionary, compulsive coping behavior.

Claudia Black (1979) considers that most children in alcoholic families adjust to the family through roles they assume in order to survive. She has identified three specific roles. By assuming responsibility for self and other siblings, the *responsible one* provides stability in the often chaotic family environment. The *adjuster* functions to reduce the amount of stress the family is experiencing. The *placater* seeks to make the other family members comfortable.

Sharon Wegscheider-Cruse (1981) has also worked extensively with members of alcoholic families. She can probably be credited with assigning the survival roles of family hero, scapegoat, mascot, and lost child to different members of the chemically dependent family system.

The Chemically Dependent Person

Contrary to what is generally believed, particularly by many affected family members, the chemically dependent person is experiencing a considerable amount of pain and shame. However, the recognition that the use behavior is responsible often eludes him or her. As the disease progresses, this person loses more and more personal control, not only of actual usage but also of behavior. As a result, the person internalizes tremendous feelings of shame, guilt, inadequacy, fear, and loneliness. To continue functioning, and in an attempt to reconcile the unreality of what is being perceived with the reality of what is actually occurring, the dependent necessarily must take on defensive behaviors and characteristics. Central to the disease, of course, are denial, rationalization, and minimization. Other defenses that the dependent often displays are irrational anger, charm, rigidity, grandiosity, perfectionism, social withdrawal, threats, hostility, and depression.

Probably most significant to the family's adaptation to the dependency is the process of projection, or of attempting to place on others the responsibility for using and for the family's problems. The projection temporarily relieves some of the dependent's internal stress. At a conscious level, the dependent is generally not aware of his or her own increasing dysfunction and its impact on the family. However, the dependent does become aware of the more obvious increasing problems with the family or specific members. The only recognizable reactionary recourse for the dependent is to assign responsibility to the individual or individuals exhibiting the problem behavior. This not only dismisses the dependent's own sense of responsibility but provides further rationalization to continue using. However, because this survival mechanism lacks personal insight, the dependent continues to experience more pain which, in turn, produces even more unconscious projection.

Codependent

The codependent role is taken by the type of person commonly called the "enabler." In a booklet from the Johnson Institute (Johnson, 1986), an enabler is characterized as a person who "reacts in such a way as to shield the dependent from experiencing the full impact of the harmful consequences" of the disease. As a result, the dependent person loses any opportunity to gain what is needed most—insight regarding the severity of the chemical dependency.

I tend to see the role of the codependent as somewhat distinct from an enabler. Although codependents are enablers, other people outside the family can enable the dependent and yet not be codependent. For example, an enabler may be the coworker who covers up mistakes or extended breaks, or the employer who excuses absences because the dependent does such a good job when he is there. An enabler may be a friend who won't confront drug-related inappropriate behavior, or the policeman who drives an intoxicated person home instead of issuing a citation. Enabling is anything done to protect the chemically dependent person from suffering the consequences of, or makes allowances for, his or her behavior. Enabling does not necessarily require an ongoing relationship. Codependency, in contrast, is manifested in a relationship with an addict or a dysfunctional person.

The codependent is the person closest to the chemically dependent person and is usually the first family member to react dysfunctionally. This role is most often taken by the spouse, but it can also be taken by a parent or another sibling. The codependent becomes highly vulnerable and reactive to the developing defenses of the dependent. Just as the dependent cannot comprehend the increasing consequences of use, so does the codependent's protective measures and excuse making for the dependent block recognition of the reality of the dependency. Their rationalizations support each other's misunderstanding of the problem. Both the dependent and the codependent are engaged in a successful self-deception that allows the disease to remain hidden and to progress toward more serious stages. Furthermore, they both become victims of the disease. Codependency is covered more fully later in this chapter.

Family Hero

Generally the family hero is the oldest child in the family and works in close alliance with the codependent to maintain the family homeostasis.

This family member sees and hears more of what is really happening in the family than the other children, and feels most responsible for the family pain. By attempting to improve the family situation, the hero fills the self-worth needs of both the dependent person and the codependent. The family conveys the basic message that the hero is very special. Realizing that personal achievement provides some joy and pride to both parents, the hero strives all the harder, hoping that enough achievement will alleviate all the family pain.

This individual quickly learns to anticipate and interpret the wishes and needs of others. After all, being responsive and helpful to others is not only attractive, but results in a great many compliments. There is no awareness that the guiding influence in most of the hero's decisions is the external behavior of the chemically dependent person.

The hero is the child who will often excel in most personal endeavors and be involved in activities to gain personal recognition. This is the one child the family can be proud of and who is perceived as being an example of how well the family is functioning. Unfortunately, no amount of achievement ever seems adequate. As the family demands more and more achievement, the feeling of internalized inadequacy negates any obvious success.

Because the others in the system are locked behind their own masks of external behavior, the hero never shares in the pleasure of direct communication. With the double message of feeling unimportant, yet being special, the hero is left to make meaning out of a contradictory world. His or her own internalized feelings of pain and confusion are disguised by overachievement, superresponsibility, working hard for approval, and perfectionism. The hero typically develops an independent lifestyle away from the family.

The hero is likely to grow up to marry an alcoholic and assume the role of enabler. Not surprisingly, adulthood will find the hero being a workaholic and living under a lot of stress. Working in the service of others and putting the needs of others before those of self becomes second nature. It is not unusual for the hero to enter one of the helping professions. Because the family never took advantage of any superior insights into dealing with the family crises, perhaps others can benefit from these talents. Unfortunately, the price to be paid in this role is excessive activity, exhaustion, perfectionism, and the lonely search for some appreciation and approval.

Scapegoat

The scapegoat is the visible tip of the iceberg of the stress experienced by the family. This is the problem child. The disruptive behavior of the scapegoat demands urgent, fast attention because, added to other family crises, this new stress takes too much effort. In fact, the stress created by the dysfunction has become such a part of their lifestyle that the individual and family energy loss is not even noticed. The hero's role in the system appears to be well defined and is evidenced by good performance. The scapegoat cannot afford to look at the pain created by the family's dysfunction. To do so makes the scapegoat feel helpless because the enabler's and hero's failed efforts show that nothing can be done about it. Although he or she is expected to contribute to the family, the scapegoat's competition with the hero makes contribution impossible.

There is a certain relief for a child to receive direct communication, however reprimanding, belittling, or hostile it may be. The direct message from the family is that the scapegoat's disruptive and destructive behavior is responsible for the family's chaos. This naturally assigns some importance and power to the role. The family members do not realize that their concentration on this new focus in the family brings them some distraction and relief from the stress of the chemical dependency.

The scapegoat is keenly aware of the manipulative communication of the enabler and the hero with the chemically dependent person, and considers them dishonest. However, any criticism of the system or the behavior of others results in being accused of not caring about the balance or welfare of the family. Being critical places the scapegoat in the position of being disloyal to the family. Unable to "get in," the scapegoat learns early that defiance is a good cover for internalized feelings of hurt and inadequacy. The rejection of being thought of as disloyal, compounded by jealousy felt toward the hero, are the main components of his or her internalized hurt.

The scapegoat's reaction is silent anger turned inward. When anger is directed inward, it produces pain of such intensity that it demands some relief and relief can be achieved only by the continual acting out. Eventually, as a protection against the intense pain and anger, feelings become frozen. Little does the family realize that they share this same hurt and anger with the scapegoat. Instead of having any sense of commonality with the rest of the family, however, the scapegoat feels rejected and withdraws from the family. Sometimes there is the desire to make the ultimate withdrawal—suicide.

Characteristic defensive behaviors for the scapegoat are self-pity, strong peer values, defiance, and hostility. Alcohol or drug use and delinquent behavior usually begin at an early age. The scapegoat grows up with a tremendous amount of internalized anger directed toward self and others. As an adult, his or her hostile behavior, resulting from the internalized anger and resentment, creates difficulty in holding a job and forming relationships. Chemical dependency and an involvement in criminal activity are not uncommon for this individual.

Mascot

The mascot is the member who at least tries to bring some fun and humor into the family and usually functions as the family pet. The purpose of the role is to distract and to relieve tension. The mascot must work hard and fast to do almost anything to secure attention. Perhaps in the middle of a heated altercation between the parents, the child destined to become the family mascot unintentionally does something and the parents break up in laughter. The mascot very quickly learns that the best way to diffuse tension is with laughter.

In the chemically dependent family, which is so preoccupied with its problems, it is difficult to compete for attention. The achievement-oriented actions of the hero and the disruptive behavior of the scapegoat can demand the family's full attention. The mascot manages to be noticed by clowning, making attempts at switching the subject, and displaying various forms of nervous humor. Commanding the center of attention provides some sense of personal control, offers more order in the chaotic environment, and creates good feelings inside. Other family members reward the humor with laughter. It is difficult to be seriously critical of someone when laughing at their antics. The mascot accepts the laughter as approval and can thereby survive the pain. The humor successfully masks all inner painful feelings.

Characteristic defensive behaviors are hyperactivity, charm, being super cute, and doing anything to get a laugh or be the center of attention. As a result, the mascot is on the way toward building a lifestyle for avoiding pain through humorous control. Unfortunately, the mascot pays the high price of loneliness, knowing that no one really knows the real person. No one sees the tears behind the clown mask, or senses the panic the mascot feels when not the center of attention, or perceives the mascot's sadness at the lack of intimacy. Most people don't take the mascot too seriously because they believe that he or she has only a limited understanding of anything too serious.

This child develops into an immature and insecure adult with the inability to seriously recognize and express feelings. The mascot continues being the clown to mask extremely low self-esteem. He or she may make a good comedian. I personally suspect that many professional comedians who "joke" about their family as part of their routine may have evolved from this role. They may be unable to express deep feelings of compassion and sensitivity toward others, for fear of ridicule and rejection. The mascot commonly makes attempts at intimacy with inappropriate humor or self-deprecation and covers up painful feelings of inadequacy with humor. The mascot's anger at being unable to relate true feelings creates an uncontrollable rage toward self. He or she sometimes manifests this rage by behavior inviting others to inflict abuse, as if it were punishment well deserved.

Lost Child

The lost child has much in common with the scapegoat. Both feel insignificant and unimportant within the family. Both learn quickly that the family spends its prime energy and creativity in protecting the dependent person. However, the lost child finds it easier to become a loner. This becomes a tremendous relief to the family. This child never creates a need to worry. The family inadvertently rewards the avoidance of stress by complimenting the withdrawal, expressing relief at having a quiet child that causes no trouble. The lost child opts more and more for building a private world and going through life on the fringes of the family pain rather than becoming involved in it.

Although liked by everyone in the family, this child's isolation often results in being ignored by other members. The child is not given certain information, suffers broken promises, or is actually excluded from some family activities. The hurt prompts a search for short-term relief in solitary pleasure, such as continuously watching TV, reading, listening to music, drugs, object love, eating, and/or living in a fantasy world. Suffering pain and loneliness, particularly in attempting interpersonal relationships, is the norm for this child.

For this child to survive in the family requires that he or she become independent. The family communication may consist of double messages, but in his or her fantasy life the lost child is in charge of putting things in order. Childhood dreams of having the perfect family sharpen the imagination to a point where the definition between fantasy and reality becomes blurred. Some lost children relate more easily with their imaginary friends or stuffed animals than with real friends.

Having learned not to make close connections in the family carries over into adult personal life. In trying to establish a relationship, the lost child feels inadequate because of his or her inability to communicate. In fact, much confusion arises over friendship and sexual involvement, disagreements and arguments, possessions and materialism. This confusion leads to many mistakes of judgment. The hurt of starting over in a relationship again and again makes being alone look very welcome and secure. Others have rewarded avoidance so often that the lost child knows that the rage he or she experiences may not be expressed. Quiet avoidance has become a lifestyle for this person.

As an adult, this person is likely superindependent, a loner, quiet, and perhaps still involved in a fantasy life. The role of the lost child lays the groundwork for some serious adult problems, such as being under- or overweight, physical and emotional distances, promiscuity, sexual identity problems, or sexual dysfunction. There is also a likelihood of being extremely attached to things and being materialistic. Because developing a fantasy life has been a major factor in growing up, the lost child can be highly creative.

Although these roles are fairly distinct, family members can switch roles when the family needs to fill a vacant part of a triangle. For example, the hero is a natural to step into the codependent role. However, although these roles are characteristic of alcoholic or chemically dependent families, they are not necessarily fully played out in every family. Both Black (1981) and Wegscheider (1981) have nevertheless concluded that children in dependent homes learn to not feel, not trust, and not talk about the family's problems. As a result, they can shut down emotionally and, as adults, have difficulty bonding and trusting and have significant problems with psychosocial adjustment.

In assigning these labels to people, I feel a note of caution is necessary. Making a connection with one of these roles can be advantageous in helping an individual discover a framework for beginning or developing a journey toward growth and autonomy. However, I have often seen an over-identification with the victim role. It is important to remember that all family members, including the dependent, are victims of the dependency. However, continuing to assume the victim role negates individual responsibility for change. A child rarely has a choice afforded him or her for avoiding abuse. As an adult, a person can only remain a victim and chained to the past so long as that is allowed. It becomes a matter of personal responsibility for an adult to work through the painful issues and let go of the past. To not do so keeps the adult in bondage to the past and to those who inflicted the pain.

CODEPENDENCY

Codependency is a fairly recent and common term that has rather frequently and loosely been used, and overused, to label many people with certain characteristics. I once heard a group member accuse another, who was setting up chairs for a group, of being codependent. In another instance, a person offering to help out another who had recently undergone major surgery was described as being codependent. Deriving pleasure from doing for or helping others is not necessarily the same as codependency.

Wegscheider-Cruse (1985) refers to codependency as a specific condition characterized by preoccupation and extreme dependence on a person or object. Eventually, this dependence becomes a pathological condition that affects the codependent in all other relationships. Gorski (1992) describes codependency as a "cluster of symptoms or maladaptive behavior changes associated with living in a committed relationship with either a chemically dependent person or a chronically dysfunctional person either as children or adults" (p. 15). Although definitions may differ somewhat, the common elements are that the codependent person is overinvolved with the dependent, is obsessed with attempting to control the behavior of the dependent, is inclined to achieve a sense of self-worth from the approval of others, and tends to make personal sacrifices for the dependent.

People raised in a chemically dependent atmosphere share fairly recognizable traits and patterns. Cermak (1986) has suggested that a codependent individual might be considered as any adult who has voluntarily remained in any dysfunctional relationship, at a considerable sacrifice of self, for at least two years without making any positive change. Children obviously can become codependent adults as the result of being raised in a dysfunctional family. Unfortunately, children rarely have the opportunity to get help for themselves while under their parents' care, nor are they able to easily leave the family. It's not at all unusual for codependent adults to feel as though they are trapped in a relationship, but the children are most certainly trapped.

There is currently no universally accepted definition of codependency. Most members of chemically dependent families, however, do exhibit a recognizable and predictable pattern of traits. Timmen Cermak characterizes codependency as a collection of maladaptive personality traits, internalized from distorted patterns experienced in childhood, that result in maladaptive relationship formation in adulthood. Codependence has marked traits of several personality disorders.

Cermak (1986) suggests that there should be specific DSM-IV diagnostic criteria for a Codependent Personality Disorder. These criteria would address the necessity to control self and others, assuming responsibility for meeting others' needs, diffuse boundaries, enmeshed relationships with the chemically dependent or other personality disordered individuals. In addition he has identified several behavioral possibilities, including that of remaining "in a primary relationship with an active substance abuser for at least two years without seeking outside help" (p. 11).

Cermak has also subgrouped codependence into specific variants. The *Martyrs* sacrifice themselves because they feel they have no choice in how they live and that any alternatives are too frightening. The *Persecutors* blame others for their misery. *The coconspirators* are not willing to recognize the chemical dependency and its related consequences, and undermine the dependent's attempts at recovery. The *Drinking* (or *Drugging*) *Partners* feel that to join with the dependent in using permits a closer connection and provides the opportunity to better control the dependent's use. And finally, the *Apathetic Codependents* have given up and simply stopped feeling and caring about much in life.

John Bradshaw (1988) considers codependency to be a symptom of abandonment. Abandonment, as he has defined it, includes neglect, abuse, and enmeshment. Bradshaw's definition, "Co-dependence is a loss of one's inner reality and an addiction to outer reality" (p. 166), very briefly assesses what therapists see in working with chemically dependent families.

The multigenerational transmission of codependent traits and patterns can most assuredly be observed. No matter how unsatisfactory children considered their parents' relationship, or how abusively parents might have treated them, they will very likely repeat the same patterns in their own primary relationships. Specific behavior manifested in the new relationship or with parenting of their children may be somewhat different, but the patterns remain the same.

Codependency most noticeably manifests itself in the individual's need to control people and situations either directly or manipulatively. The person feels an almost consuming need to assume responsibility for another's emotional well-being and decision making and for being a perpetual caretaker. Nearly always these "good acts" sacrifice the self. The person also tends to continue to subject oneself to emotional, physical, or sexual abuse.

The codependent role is played out rather noticeably in the chemically dependent family. The codependent internalizes the dependent's increasing projection as growing feelings of guilt and self-blame, which are characterized as a series of "if onlys": "If only I had been more responsive to his needs," "If only I had been more intimate," "If only I had been a better lover." Eventually the codependent becomes convinced that he or she is responsible for the dependent's intoxication and behavior. Feeling responsible then creates the belief that the dependent's drinking or drug use can be controlled by reactive behaviors: "If I caused it, I must be able to cure it." This conviction requires the codependent to employ a variety of tactics to reverse or correct the actions he or she believes were responsible. Of course, because the codependent cannot identify just what particular behavior "caused" the dependent's use, all kinds of irrational behavior ensue. Attempts at control may involve checking up on the dependent when away from home, canceling social events, disposing of liquor or drug supplies, taking over some of the dependent's responsibilities, or making excuses to others for the intoxicated behavior.

All attempts at control, however, are futile. The continued experience of failure contributes even more to the codependent's diminishing self-worth. The declining self-worth results in emotional isolation and loneliness. It is important to realize what is happening to this person at an emotional level. As the internalized feelings of pain, anger, low self-worth, and loneliness increase, the codependent's reactions to the dependent become more and more compulsive. The dependent's chemical use is interpreted as an outward display of the enabler's internal guilt and feeling of inadequacy.

In other words, the codependent's self-worth is tied directly to the dependent's chemical use. The more the dependent uses, the more the codependent feels responsible, guilty, inadequate, and powerless. The only way for this person to feel any positive self-worth is to try to make sure the dependent's chemical use does not get out of control. The internalized conviction that something can be done to control the dependent's use, or make it go away, becomes obsessive. All attempts at manipulation and control, of course, are doomed to fail, because the codependent is trying to control the uncontrollable. With each failure the codependent's self-worth diminishes even further, which triggers even more desperate attempts to control. This continues on in a vicious cycle as both the dependent and the codependent become increasingly alienated and dysfunctional. Eventually, the codependent can become incapable of achieving the emotional stability and insight needed to deal with the disease in any effective manner.

ADULT CHILDREN OF ALCOHOLICS: CHARACTERISTICS

A number of traits or characteristics have been identified in adult children of alcoholics. Obviously, not all adult children have all these characteristics, but most possess some of them. To understand how these traits have developed, consider the complex dynamics involved in the background of such people. Their survival roles, adopted to avoid pain, have led to lack of self-identity and confusion in relating with others. Unrealistic fantasies about what life would be like if their parent or parents were sober are mixed up with the chaotic reality of mixed messages and inconsistencies to which they were subjected while growing up. Overt denial of unpleasant realities, coverups, broken promises, and inconsistencies have been basic to the family system.

As children they were never good enough, never did things right, and were constantly being criticized. Immersed in such chaos, childhood was simply not much fun. They have no frame of reference for what a healthy, intimate relationship can be. As children they learned to take charge of their environment, as they envisioned their particular roles, and to trust only themselves. They translated the confused messages as being conditional love, which says, "I don't love you when you're bad." Unconditional love says, "I don't like your behavior, but I love you." As children, socializing for them was difficult, so they did not develop the social skills necessary to feel comfortable or to be a part of a group. Fear, insecurity, and the lack of social skills kept them from forming adequate relationships. Hopes, wishes, and plans were often set aside or aborted either because the family did not provide support or they themselves lacked the ability to get beyond the family chaos to fulfill them.

With this kind of childhood existence, it can be expected that the adult has formulated ineffective traits for living. Not having had the opportunity to attain good social skills, and having to guess at what is normal, adult children often have difficulty with intimate relationships. They deeply fear abandonment or rejection, and vacillate between feeling loved one day and rejected the next. Claudia Black (1979) considers that the primary problem facing adult children of alcoholics is maintenance of intimate relationships. Their sense of urgency in the relationship can make their mate feel smothered. They have a tendency to be extremely loyal in the relationship, even if there is evidence that their loyalty is undeserved. This "loyalty" is related to their fear and insecurity in the relationship. Because forming relationships is so difficult for them, once it is established they tend to make it permanent despite all odds.

There is no way to meet the standards of perfection they have internalized from childhood, so adult children tend to judge themselves harshly and be extremely demanding of themselves. They have difficulty separating self from their work. Personal identity comes from what they do and how well they do it, not from who they are. They are often controlling, rigid, lacking in spontaneity, and overreactive to changes over which they have no control. Although they may have great ideas and develop wonderful plans, they often procrastinate and have difficulty completing projects. Unconsciously, they are aware that if a project is not completed they can't be criticized for doing it wrong.

I believe it is important to remember that most of the literature available on children of alcoholics seems to be based on clinical observation. Therefore, clinicians are likely to see only those who come in for help. Although there seems to be no doubt that children from chemically dependent homes are vulnerable and at risk for severe trauma, some of these children may suffer little, if any, adverse affects. The degree of risk for children raised in chemically dependent homes depends a great deal, I am certain, on the severity of the parent's dependency, the ages of the children at various points, and whether or not the parents were abusive. I know of some adults who have no apparent psychological or emotional problems and report having fond memories of their father who was a "happy and lovable drunk." In addition, some individuals raised in dysfunctional families appear to have great resiliency and reach adulthood with no significant emotional problems.

Werner (1986) conducted a longitudinal study of 49 children from alcoholic homes born on the island of Kauai, Hawaii. Although the majority were reared in poverty and received little or no emotional support and educational stimulation in the home, 59 percent of these children at age 18 had no psychosocial problems. Werner found that those children who appeared resilient to the long-term effects of parental alcoholism shared certain characteristics. They had positive attention from the parents, possessed at least average intelligence and good communication skills, were achievement oriented, and were responsible and caring toward others. In addition, they had a positive self-concept and believed they could take charge of their lives and accomplish things on their own initiative.

According to Dunkel (1993), most of the research conducted on adult children of alcoholics has been short term and has not fully examined all the variables to conclusively ascertain that ACOAs are a unique group. Many problems characteristic of children from chemically dependent homes appear in adults who present psychological problems and who come from other dysfunctional family systems.

West and Prinz (1987) also consider that other factors may increase the probability that short- and long-term psychological, social, and physical problems may ensue for children raised in chemically dependent homes. Specifically, West and Prinz recognize that chemically dependent families do seem to have higher divorce rates, more family conflict, more parental psychopathology, economic factors, physical abuse and neglect, and birth complications. Any one or a combination of these factors, aside from or in addition to the chemical abuse, could produce problems for children.

I believe that it is also significant, although not usually recognized by the individual, that a good many chemically dependent people, once having achieved stabilized recovery, have a crucial need to work on their own codependency patterns related to the family of origin. Not to do so can drastically impair the adult's full potential for personal growth and place that person at high risk for relapse or finding themselves enveloped in another addiction or compulsive behavior.

EXERCISES

1. If you know people who have been raised in a chemically dependent family, identify the particular family roles they played or play.
2. Describe five types of behavior that might be considered typical for a codependent person.
3. Considering the particular functions performed by each of the children in the chemically dependent family, what kind of adult strengths can you envision as having been achieved by
   a. the family hero
   b. the scapegoat
   c. the mascot
   d. the lost child

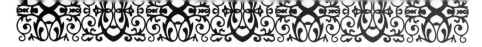

Chapter Nine

Family Assessment

Making an accurate and objective assessment of problems that actually exist in a family can, at least initially, be confusing and demanding. Each family member coming into treatment has a different view of what is going on within the family and who is responsible. Typically, a considerable amount of blame and self-blame is handed about among the members as they each try to say what they see as wrong with the family. Keep in mind that each individual is coming from his or her own reality and must be considered within that reality, even though obviously that reality may be somewhat skewed. Therefore, the counselor needs to elicit each person's perception of what he or she considers the problem to be. It is also important to learn from each of them what he or she believes has created and sustained the problem and what attempts, individually and collectively, have been made to correct it. Even when agreeing that a specific problem exists, various members will likely have different perceptions of the problem and its cause.

Family members who claim they have no idea of what the problem or concern is all about, or even that one exists, usually do have some idea, and are just not expressing it for one reason or another. Family members generally make some assumptions about the "cause" of their problems, however erroneous those assumptions may be. There may be, and usually is, more than one problem in the family. It's not at all unusual for people to come to therapy only when the family situation has become extremely complex and completely out of hand. Sometimes at least one member of the family has moved around from therapist to therapist seeking to either be "fixed" or to find out how to "fix" other family members.

Quite often the initial motive for parents seeking help is to solve problems with one or more of the children. However, the children's problems are usually generated by a dysfunctional family system. Therefore, exploring the system dynamics can help in more accurately assessing the child's situation. In most dysfunctional families, secrets are the norm. Issues such as physical or sexual abuse and chemical dependency have likely been enveloped in family denial for so long they are not quickly acknowledged by family members. Exploring the family's boundaries is crucial in this regard. Where adequate boundaries are lacking, whether only between two members or the entire family, and heavy enmeshment is indicated, the chances of finding incest are greater. Incest may be perpetrated by an older sibling as well as by an adult member. In many instances, incest is committed by a grandparent or another member of the extended family.

The sometimes chaotic initial encounter with the family can make it extremely difficult for the therapist to sort through all the problems presented. It is also likely that individual family members will seek to draw the therapist into the family's dysfunction. They may want the therapist to take sides, to share in the anxiety, or to give advice on how to find an immediate solution. Successful therapy depends on getting assumptions and issues out in the open so that they can be accurately assessed and dealt with. It is imperative that the therapist maintain emotional autonomy and not get hooked into the system. To the degree that the therapist is emotionally mature and has resolved his or her own personal family-of-origin issues, he or she will be able to remain autonomous and work effectively with the family.

The chronicity and progression of chemical dependency make it a core issue for families. Whether working with the entire family or with only one member, the assessment should include an appraisal of any family member's involvement with alcohol and/or other drugs, and the frequency of use. Any indication that chemical dependency is an issue for one or more of the family members needs to result in a referral to a chemical dependency specialist for assessment and treatment recommendations. If the fact of chemical dependency is established, treatment for it should be an initial consideration for that person. Family members should be encouraged to get involved with the family component of that treatment process as well.

Often a family's need for treatment doesn't present itself until one of the members is involved in chemical dependency treatment. In that instance, the chemical dependency specialist should strongly encourage the family's concurrent involvement in treatment with the chemically dependent, wherein they can become informed about chemical dependency and its related family consequences. A referral to a family therapist after that involvement is necessary for the entire family. Obviously a number of issues must be addressed to begin restoring a more functional family life.

SPECIFIC ISSUES RELATED TO CHEMICAL DEPENDENCY

Steinglass's (1987) incorporation of the family systems approach into the dynamics of alcoholic families addresses specific issues related to chemical dependency. The family's progression of maladaptive behavior coincides with the progression of the disease. Identifying the degree of involvement or the stage of addiction can provide a clue as to the degree of accommodation or adaptation the family has made to the illness. This information is crucial to making an accurate determination of a course of treatment for the chemically dependent as well as for the other family members.

In working with the families, it is important to know not only what accommodation the family has made to incorporate the chronic condition of chemical dependency as a part of its identity, but also to what extent the family has endured or is willing to endure its consequences.

During the early stage of addiction, very little accommodation has been made by family members. Nor has much adaptation been made to their respective roles. However, the family has expended considerable energy in their concern about current use and in their unconscious attempt to prevent repetition of heavy use. The anger and resentment that family members feel is not always readily evident, nor openly expressed. Because this stage of dependency is generally characterized by denial and minimization by the entire family, dependency is usually not recognized as the primary family problem. Family members typically make excuses for the dependent regarding behavior and incidents related to drinking and drug use.

By the middle stage of dependency, the family has made considerable accommodation and adaptation to the chemical dependency. Family roles have been compromised and shifted. Reactions to the dependent vary among family members. One individual may take on more responsibility; another may seek to protect the dependent by a variety of enabling behaviors. Still another may isolate him- or herself because of embarrassment or fear of recrimination. Some members may be accusatory and assign blame for all the family's problems to the dependent. And finally, others may still deny that a problem exists. During this time one can begin to see the formation of the rather distinct survival roles typical of the chemically dependent family.

By the late stage of dependency, adaptive roles have become fairly rigid. There may be a family conspiracy against the dependent, seeking to exclude him or her from normal family activities. The family may be feeling a great deal of guilt and shame, and yet appear to have resigned itself to the family's seemingly hopeless condition.

Active use of alcohol and drugs disturbs memory function, mood, cognition, sleep, and interactional behavior. Therefore, another important issue to consider in observing the family is how the members have learned to communicate nonverbally through facial expression, body posture, and voice inflection. Because use patterns often are cyclical, behavior during periods of intoxication may contrast with behavior during sobriety. For instance, abusive behavior or irresponsibility may only manifest itself during periods of intoxication. Family members may show corresponding reactionary behavior patterns, such as emotional withdrawal or rescuing the dependent during periods of intoxication. Chemical dependency has a high degree of predictability, and remarkably consistent patterns of behavior can be observed during periods of intoxication. In the family, predictable patterns of responsive behavior associated with the chemical use can also be expected. Families with chemically dependent members constitute highly complex behavior systems. Some families also have a remarkable tolerance for stress. They can make quite creative bursts of adaptive behavior in response to the dependent's use.

One cannot consistently characterize the chemically dependent person with any simple formula that considers only cultural factors and the complexities of use behavior and patterns. Neither can a typical chemically dependent family be defined. There is considerable variation, not only with usual sociodemographic and biological characteristics, but also with dynamic and behavioral aspects of life. To really understand the addictive family system, consideration must also be given to the multi-generational nature of the relationship between chemical dependency and the family.

As Steinglass (1987) has identified, very different consequences of chemical dependency can be experienced by different families:

1. In one family, chemical dependency may be associated with a coping style centered around an attempt to isolate the affected individual. This is an attempt to protect other family members from possible consequences of the behavior while intoxicated.
2. In another family, the use-affected behavior may go virtually unnoticed by other family members.
3. Another family might view the chemical dependency as inevitable, considering it predetermined, a built-in feature of life. This view is usually closely linked to the family's cultural or ethnic values.
4. Still another family might be fully aware of the consequences that the dependency imposes on family life but still be helpless to effectively cope with it.

In many instances, family members, usually with good intentions, tend to make matters worse by reacting in ways that amplify rather than diminish problems. As discussed earlier, for many families chemical dependency can become a central organizing principle around which family life is structured.

Family dysfunction has a definable course of development or progression, just as does chemical dependency. However, there are a number of variables in consumption practices and behavior of the dependent and in the family's reaction and adaptation to them, so established long-term patterns result in different life histories for different families. The counselor must determine how closely and consistently the use pattern of the dependent individual fits the characteristics of family organization.

Observation of the family dynamics should, according to Steinglass (1987), consider four basic questions:

1. Have chemical dependency and its related behaviors become the central organizing principle around which the family has structured its life?
2. To what extent has the introduction of chemical dependency into family life altered the homeostasis between growth and regulation, and has the family shifted to placing emphasis on short-term stability at the expense of long-term growth?
3. What type of changes have occurred in family functioning and regulatory behaviors as the family has gradually accommodated to the demands of the dependency?
4. In what manner have the regulatory behaviors been altered to profoundly influence the overall shape of family growth and development?

By analyzing the responses to these questions a determination can be made as to how severely the family has been affected by chemical dependency.

OTHER CRITICAL ISSUES

A number of other issues frequently occur in chemically dependent families. A diligent attempt should be made to ascertain the existence and the extent of any of them. Also, a determination should be made as to the frequency of specific issues and whether any particular situation occurs only during occasions of chemical use or at times other than active use.

Emotional Abuse

Emotional abuse may consist of name calling, derogatory or caustic remarks, criticism, put-downs, ridicule, "the silent treatment," or emotional withdrawal. Any type of verbal or nonverbal behavior intended to demean a person is emotional abuse. Although not physically injurious, emotional abuse can cause serious psychological damage, particularly to the self-esteem of a developing child. Consistent emotional abuse results in an internalization, for both adults and children, of a poor self-concept, feelings of unworthiness, and of being unloved.

Domestic Violence

Domestic violence takes many forms, from a back-hand slap or shove to actual beating with or without some object. It not only has the potential for severe physical harm, or even death, but for serious psychological damage. Many victims don't even consider that the slap or shove or arm grabbing is abusive. Most victims have become convinced, by their abuser, that they have done something to deserve the assault. Regardless of the abuse level, it will only escalate over time, and the recipient must takes steps to protect him- or herself and other potential victims in the family. Although most reported incidences concern men battering women and children, some men are victims of battering. Particularly if the abuse is serious, either the victims must be removed to safety or the perpetrator removed from the home.

Sexual Abuse

Sexual abuse of a spouse is not uncommon in the chemically dependent family. Between marital partners it can consist of withholding of sex, using sex as a means to attain something, or an actual forced sexual act. Probably the most psychologically damaging abuse to children is incest. Sexually abused children can't hope to reach adulthood without having suffered considerable emotional trauma and the acquisition of a multitude of misconceptions about intimacy and sex. On the discovery of any level of sexual abuse, immediate action should be initiated to remove the perpetrator from the home. The victimized children will require extensive specialized treatment in an attempt to overcome their trauma.

Abandonment

The possibility of abandonment of the children also requires attention. Obviously small children being left alone or with others and neglect of physical needs by the parents constitutes abandonment. But abandonment can also take the form of emotional distancing. Sometimes the marital relationship is so enmeshed that consideration of the children becomes secondary to the couple's relationship needs and closeness. Sometimes one parent can become so preoccupied with the other parent's chemical use that the children's needs are disregarded. There are also parents who, because their own emotional needs are not being met in the marital relationship, become triangulated with one of the children to the exclusion of the others.

Other Illnesses or Conditions

A member with a serious physical or mental illness can also significantly influence a family's functioning. It's not unusual in the chemically dependent family to find one or more other members with an eating disorder, drug use, or other compulsive behavior. All these factors can seriously compound problems already associated with the chemical dependency. The more dysfunctional the family, the less able members are to make adequate adjustment to any of these situations.

In addition, it is important to explore significant behavioral problems with each child. Children who are close together in age or the same sex share a natural basis for competition. Special children (such as disabled, extraordinary, or adopted) can also influence family positioning. How the children relate to one another and to the parents, and how each perceives his or her position in the family, is important information. Note and explore any unusual circumstances, such as family deaths or other losses, traumatic events, geographical relocations, significant career changes, and an adult returning to school.

BIRTH ORDER OF THE CHILDREN

Birth order of the children can be a significant factor in any family's functioning. Each child has to find a place for him- or herself in the family, and characteristics of its chronological placement in the family, theoretically, in and of itself can force a child into a particular role.

An only child has a unique position in that he or she holds both the youngest and oldest place in the family. This child tends to combine serious, overresponsible, and adultlike behavior and to not allow the childlike charm of self show through. Often a high expectation is placed on the only child to always maintain loyalty to the family. Many only children among adults with whom I've worked disclosed that they functioned in each of the previously identified roles of the chemically dependent family at one time or another in growing up.

The oldest child tends to become more adultlike than younger siblings. He or she is often rational, analytic, and responsible, and identifies more closely with the family's established values and themes. Many performance expectations are placed on this child. As a result, he or she will, despite evidence to the contrary, often have a sense of never performing well enough. A son is often expected to be the family standard bearer. The expected role of an oldest daughter is usually that of nurturer. This child is a natural to fall into the role of the family hero.

The middle child has greater difficulty finding a place in the family because he or she is squeezed both from the top and bottom of birth order. Middle children may be the least likely to feel constrained by family norms and to develop parallel peer networks. They generally are better socially skilled than the other siblings, but have difficulty developing self-identity. They may be conscious that something is wrong in the family but not be able to figure out just what it is, and so will absorb the family's emotional issues. This child may fulfill the lost child role in the chemically dependent family.

The youngest child has a unique position. The last child represent an issue of loss for the parents. This child very often becomes rebellious and a risk taker because he or she is not as constrained by family rules as other siblings. The child may appear somewhat uninvolved with the family. In fact, this child may be very involved because he or she feels responsible for what is going on in the family and yet seems powerless to do anything about it. Reactive behavior displayed may be either disruptive or clowning, respectively, resembling the scapegoat or mascot in the chemically dependent family.

The functioning of sibling positions is not cast in cement, and different families may experience different roles. I once encountered a family of four children who all fell precisely into well-defined family roles of a chemically dependent family. In this instance, the oldest child was the scapegoat, the second oldest was the mascot, the third child was the lost child, and the youngest was the hero.

Information Gathering

To get a complete picture of a family, the counselor must begin gathering factual information and obtaining historical data concerning the presenting problems and how they interrelate with the symptomatic behavior of other members. Carefully listening to the story or stories being presented and attempting to learn fairly exact dates of when the symptoms developed or recurred can be helpful later when these data are correlated with additional information gathered. It is crucial to obtain information not only about what specific problems exist currently, but also about what patterns have developed within the nuclear family over time.

The nuclear family begins when a man and woman are married. A good way to learn the historical development of the family is to gather information about what each was doing when they met, and any previous marriages and children. The age of the parents at the time of the children's birth, the spacing and gender of the children, and how soon a child was born after the loss of another are helpful pieces of information. For instance, the arrival of a new baby shortly after the death of another child may result in one or both of the parents not bringing closure to their grief over the loss. Other information, such as educational level and previous physical or psychological problems encountered, helps develop a picture of the family system. It is also helpful to know the level of drinking or drug use and each partner's attitude toward the use at the time they began their relationship.

The easiest way to gather and sort out these data is to begin developing a genogram, which can clearly delineate individual functioning. A genogram can portray patterns of relating in symbiotic relationships, triangles, and boundaries (or lack thereof). Once the counselor has mapped the nuclear family, over time he or she can add historical information relating to the extended family. Information on the extended family should include much the same data as gathered for the nuclear family. When chemical dependency is an issue, the counselor should explore patterns in previous generations, and related family attitudes and dynamics.

CREATING A GENOGRAM

A genogram is a graphic depiction of how family members are related to one another within a single generation and from one generation to the next. It is a family map. The genogram not only involves mapping out the family structure, but is a way to record family history and determine the interplay of family relationships. It is generally considered most helpful to include at least three generations, two beyond the family with which you are working (assuming you are working with the last nuclear family).

The genogram provides a framework for exploring emotional boundaries, enmeshment, triangulations, existing conflict, and the number of current or potential relationships within the family. It graphically displays family information that can help set a clinical issue in the context of family dynamics. One can readily learn about the emotional forces existing with the family, both vertically and horizontally. Family triangulations become readily apparent. One can instantly see family members, unresolved conflict, strong family bonds, distancing, and indicators of past (and potential) chemical dependency, incest, or abuse.

The genogram is usually constructed in the first session and is updated as new information becomes available during later sessions. It thus provides an efficient clinical summary as the family "portrait" emerges, displaying patterns and recurring events that may have significance. The genogram can also be helpful in getting family members to see how patterns and family interactions have developed and what is blocking appropriate functioning for them.

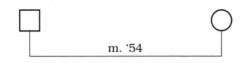

FIGURE 9-1 _____

Different clinicians use a variety of symbols in developing the genogram. Some add their own symbols. The particular symbols used are not so important as the dynamics they represent. McGoldrick and Gerson's *Genograms in Family Assessment* (1985) describes fairly standard symbols for developing a graphic display of the family.

In McGoldrick and Gerson's system, each family member is represented either by a box (for males) or a circle (for females). Family legal and biological relationships are connected by lines. Family members and emotional ties are depicted by various symbols. One would begin by indicating first the father on the left and the mother on the right with a connecting line and their year of marriage (Figure 9-1). A cohabitative relationship is depicted the same, except that the line is broken (Figure 9-2). Separation and divorces are denoted on the marriage line with a / or // respectively. Children are added below the marriage line, with the oldest on the left and moving to the right in descending order, using the symbols as shown in Figure 9-3.

Above each family member's symbol, the year of birth and death, if such is the case, are indicated. The current age or age at death is noted inside the member symbol, and the name of the individual written above or below the symbol. The symbol of a deceased family member is marked *x*, and the identified patient is marked by an inner square or circle (Figure 9-4). Other symbols that depict the emotional forces within the family system are portrayed in Figure 9-5.

To depict alcoholism or chemical dependency, I place an "A" or "CD" to the left of the individual's symbol. An "/R" after this designation indicates the person is in recovery. A family portrait, therefore, might look something like the four-generation family genogram shown in Figure 9-6.

Other important information that can be gathered about each family member is their educational level, occupation, geographical location, religious background, major relocations, career changes, major illnesses, causes of death, and ethnic background. Significant emotional events, particularly as they relate to the individuals with whom one is working,

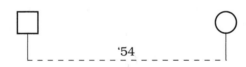

FIGURE 9-2 _____

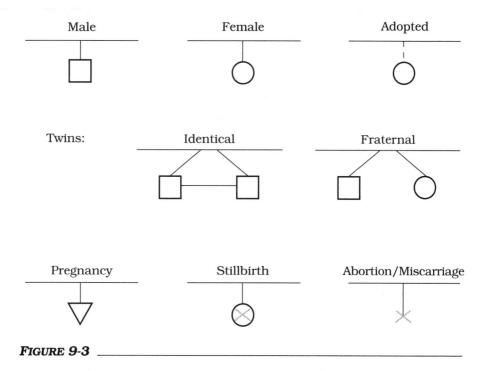

FIGURE 9-3

most definitely should be identified. Once at least part of the family structure is in place, add the symbols representing the emotional system (such as closeness, distancing, conflict, and so forth) as they pertain to the various family members. I find it helpful to use different colors to more readily differentiate the interactions.

EXERCISES

1. Describe an example of each of the four ways in which alcoholism or addiction can have different consequences for different families.
2. From the Figure 9-6 genogram, identify two or three particular patterns transmitted from one generation to another.
3. Using the genogram in Figure 9-6, describe how the relationships might have developed had some or all of them still been actively using.
4. Draft a genogram of your own immediate family.

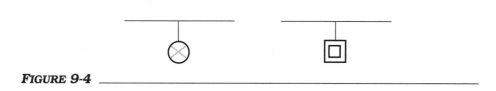

FIGURE 9-4

Conflict

Closeness

Enmeshed

Estranged/Cut Off

Rigid Boundary

Clear, Permeable Boundary

Difffuse Boundary

FIGURE 9-5

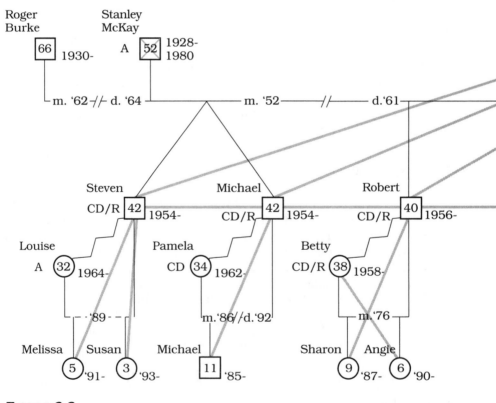

FIGURE 9-6

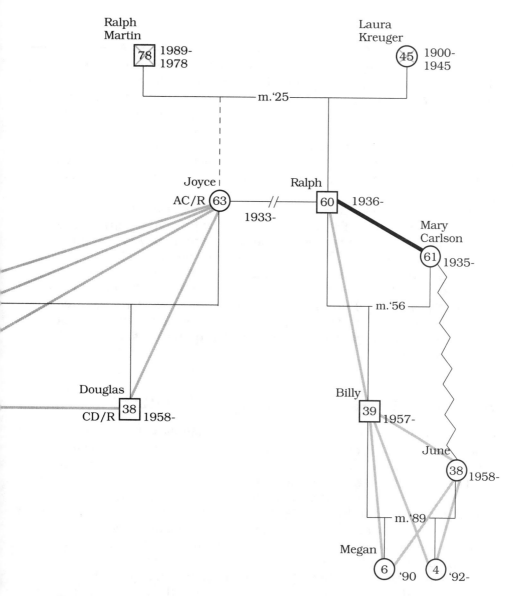

FIGURE 9-6

Chapter Ten

Working with Chemically Dependent Families

Some chemically dependent families have a tremendous capacity to withstand stress. It is possible to find them appearing, at least on the surface, fairly structurally intact and functioning somewhat competently. They may remain economically viable over time and may avoid the more serious and damaging types of family violence. They may also appear to have suffered no higher levels of anxiety and depression than the general population. However, despite all appearances, these families are quite likely leading lives compromised by exposure to chemical dependency.

Some families also can maintain long-term relationships that significantly restrict family life. Over time, the chemical dependency may have strained the family's energy and resources. However, if there is an absence of physical violence or employment problems, for instance, the family chemical dependency may not be perceived as a significant threat to survival. Even so, the impact of the disease on the fundamental aspects of family life affects families. As demonstrated earlier, the impact on the family's daily routines, rituals, and problem-solving strategies can be so profound that it shapes their entire life history.

FRAMEWORK FOR WORKING WITH FAMILIES

To work effectively with chemically dependent families, the counselor needs a conceptual framework that acknowledges all the complexities involved. Such a framework views the family as a set of interconnected individuals acting together as a unique social unit. It recognizes that the family unit, particularly in the presence of chemical dependency, has changed in a somewhat predictable fashion over time.

Once the family's major presenting issues have been sorted out and priorities have been set, a course of action must be established. Most chemically dependent families have very little, if any, understanding of chemical dependency. Family members often feel personally responsible for causing the disease and are reluctant to address those issues in fear of being further blamed by the counselor. Parents are often unwilling to accept their child's chemical dependency because they feel it reflects on their ability to parent.

It is also common for family members to believe that if the drinking or drug use ceases, all their problems will go away. Therefore, family members need to become aware of how each has enabled the dependent and contributed to the family's problems in accommodating to use-related behaviors. Simply discontinuing alcohol or drug use does not solve the family's problems. Particularly if the dependency has not yet progressed beyond the earlier stages, gaining an understanding of chemical dependency, its progression, and consequences may prompt family members to seek help in changing their reactiveness to the dependent. Even if the dependent continues to use, the family members can become able to impede the progression within the family system.

Denial and rationalization are very often more predominant with other family members than with the chemically dependent member. It's much easier to assign all responsibility and blame for the family's problems to the obvious perpetrator, to the person drinking, than to see oneself as contributing to and sustaining the problem. The counselor should enhance gentle confrontation of the denial by providing evidence of observed reactive patterns that have developed or are being sustained within the system. A genogram can provide a graphic display of patterns and role adaptations to chemical dependency, both current and in prior generations.

As previously indicated, family systems theory is basically a philosophy or a manner in which to view families and their interactional patterns. It does not offer a specific set of techniques with which to promote change. Almost any therapeutic approach can work well within the framework of the theory. The basic goal of systems theory is for each family member to achieve a higher level of functioning and emotional maturity. To do so, family members must acknowledge and address hidden conflict and secrets, dissolve triangles, redirect reactionary patterns, and establish appropriate boundaries. Furthermore, each member must come to acknowledge and change his or her contribution, not only to the family's dysfunction, but to how individual and collective response patterns have sustained the chemical dependency.

The principal challenge for the counselor in working with families is to remain detached. An underfunctioning individual can form a kind of vacuum that pulls in an overfunctioning person, and then they continue to feed on one another in a circuitous fashion. If the counselor is uncertain of his or her own beliefs and has unresolved personal issues, remaining detached and not being pulled into the family emotional system can be difficult.

In many circumstances, it may be preferable to work with only one or two members rather than the entire family. Each person who is a part of a problem, especially within the nuclear family, has some responsibility in it. However, each person can successfully work on his or her part of it, whether the others are equally motivated for treatment. Even if a couple comes in together to work on the "problem," often one partner is not motivated for treatment. The counselor can focus on the individual in whom the greatest strength seems to lie. The person in a strong role can modify his or her part in the problem more easily than the person in the weaker role. There is a good chance that a change in the reaction and behavior of the better functioning person can modify at least that part of the system. If this modification successfully alters that person's way of relating to the dependent and to the other members of the family, they too will be forced to shift and modify their positions.

The systems approach to viewing families is also effective when working with single adults. Moreover, someone physically separated from the family can be as much a part of the emotional system as someone within the home. As already discussed, every family emotional system has its roots deep in multigenerational history. That history determines its characteristics and its levels of responsible functioning. This results in an extremely complex blend of forces in which each member plays a role. Whenever any one member attempts to change a role, that change, however desirable, will disturb the old balance and provoke some resistance among other family members. As resistance to the change builds up, the resultant anxiety can be difficult for the family to deal with. Therefore, other family members are forced to alter their manner of responding to each other, whether they are inclined to do so or not.

THE COURSE OF FAMILY TREATMENT

For the family as a unit and for its members individually to achieve a higher degree of functioning and emotional maturity, a number of objectives need to be accomplished at different levels of treatment. At some point, family reconstruction and restoration of intimacy must occur. Before those issues can be successfully addressed, however, some preliminary tasks must be accomplished. The therapist's role at each phase of treatment is to help family members accomplish their various objectives.

Perhaps even before making a complete assessment of the entire family system, the counselor should appraise the severity of the chemical dependency and the impact it has had on each member. Once objectives have been established and addressed in that regard, the counselor can proceed to evaluate the obvious dynamics, boundaries, specific roles adopted, and member alliances.

In conducting a family evaluation, consider each person's feelings and sense of reality about him- or herself, and each person's position in the family. At this time the therapist might draw some preliminary conclusion as to the least and most functioning members, as well as those most amenable to treatment. A determination can also be made as to who is to be seen, whether the whole family, individually, in pairs, or as a combination of members.

Once the therapist has diagnosed chemical dependency, he or she must label it as a family problem. The next objective is to stop the drinking and/or drug use and to develop the most appropriate course of treatment for the dependent. If treatment entry for the dependent is not successful at this time, education on chemical dependency and strategy planning for an intervention may be appropriate for the family, if the family members are emotionally stable and functional enough. If the family members are not psychologically or emotionally prepared to intervene, family therapy should continue, perhaps without the dependent person. Whatever the course for the dependent, family members should deal with their own denial and arrive at some recognition of their own contribution to the problem. This can occur whether or not the dependent is amenable to treatment or willing to remain abstinent. It is crucial that family members recognize that they didn't cause the chemical dependency and that they can't control or cure it. They need to be encouraged to stop taking responsibility for the dependent so that he or she can realize the full consequences of his or her dependency.

Primary treatment should begin with basic education on chemical dependency, its progression, how it affects the family, along with the enabling behavior of family members. The counselor must also begin working on the shame and guilt associated with their belief that they caused the addiction or could somehow have prevented it, as well as on the issue of blame directed toward the dependent. Some education on effective communication and how to more appropriately respond to the dependent's behavior is crucial. These tasks generally become the focus of initial and primary treatment and can be provided by the chemical dependency specialist. Unfortunately, many families won't seek to move beyond this point.

After primary treatment, the challenge for the family becomes an attempt at regaining some degree of balance in the system, with the assistance of a family therapist. Here the focus might be on modifying family rules and defining and clarifying individual boundaries. Some degree of consistency in styles of interaction must be implemented, particularly in dealing with the children. The counselor may need to provide some basic parenting skills training at this time. Basic changes made by the adult members can, of themselves, bring about a change in the patterns and behavior of the children.

Once the family system has gained or regained some degree of balance, the objective becomes that of restoring intimacy within the relationship. The challenge here is helping family members to communicate and relate to each other directly. They must learn to appropriately recognize, express, and take ownership of their feelings. Each person must be able to request what is needed or desired from the others.

As each adult member of the family begins to interact more appropriately with each other and with the children, treatment should focus on more deeply ingrained issues arising from the family of origin. Younger children in the family also may require some additional work with specific issues, particularly if there has been a history of abuse.

As a family and as individuals, achieving a higher level of self-esteem and personal empowerment will result in each person becoming less emotionally dependent on others. Personal empowerment provides inner control for meeting one's own wants and needs and building self-confidence. Adult members need to be encouraged to reexperience and relive old, familiar patterns of the maternal and paternal families of origin. This provides the opportunity to view old family patterns in their reality, to challenge them and to attempt new patterns. Some of the original power of the parents can be released by looking at them as persons rather than roles and by honestly assessing their personal strengths and weaknesses. This provides an opportunity to determine how their parents became the way they were and to recognize their humanness. Help them recognize that, despite their dysfunction, their parents have provided them with some positive characteristics. Traits considered might be such things as work ethic, honesty, integrity, persistence, and survival.

Ongoing tasks may need to include providing assistance with the attempt to reconcile estranged members and to deal with any unfinished business from the past. Resolving issues from the family of origin and relinquishing the power of the parents can help adults move from needing acceptance of others to achieving self-acceptance and personal empowerment. Ultimately family members need to recognize and accept that changing parents and other family members is not essential to happy, successful living, but that changing oneself is.

WORKING CONSIDERATIONS

To work effectively with families, the counselor needs to be aware of a number of considerations. Steinglass (1987) has identified several factors for the counselor to keep in mind. First, symptoms in children help stabilize rocky marriages. The children's symptoms are likely to manifest in some kind of disruptive behavior. If a small symptom of the child cannot stabilize the marriage, a larger symptom or worse behavior is needed. The greater the magnitude of the marital conflict, the more severe the child's symptom. The more covert or hidden the conflict, the more a symptom is needed to stabilize the marital conflict so that it can remain hidden. Generally, if a child's symptom is eliminated, the marital conflict intensifies. However, the more openly the partners fight, the easier it is to help the family system change. Once the partners acknowledge and deal with the marital conflict, the child seldom remains symptomatic. Parents must be held responsible for their children, the contention being that a problem in a child is projected there through the mechanism of triangles.

A person's primary loyalty is nearly always with the family, even if the family is dysfunctional. The therapist must not try to condemn nor compete with someone's family. It's wise to imagine that other family members are always invisibly present in the therapy room. If the therapist condemns, belittles, or judges parents, the client may become defensive about them.

A family system operates within a present, past, and future. Each family system has its own unique history and structure as influenced by the parents, and the parents are the architects of the family. Present interactional patterns are derived from past generations and are governed by the family's hopes and goals for the future. There is certainly nothing inherently wrong in planning for the future. However, when future hopes and goals control behavior to the degree that present context is ignored, maladaptive behavior will likely result.

No ideal characteristics of all family systems exist. Each family system is as unique as each member within it. The family system grows in direct relation to the degree that the individual members have developed an internal system that allows for their own growth. A functional family allows individual growth. Likewise, there is no single, typical chemically dependent family. As Steinglass points outs, alcohol or drug use has very different implications in different families. In one family it may act as a divisive force, for example, family members try to isolate themselves from the dependent. In another family it may serve as a cohesive function; family members rally together to protect the dependent.

In addition, the level of distress and the magnitude of chemical dependency's negative consequences within a family unit are often unrelated to either the actual quantity or frequency of alcohol or drug consumption. In other words, given family-of-origin history and acceptance of use, one family might consider heavy consumption fairly normal and to be expected, whereas another family might consider it unacceptable. The actual impact of chemical dependency on the family may be largely determined by characteristics of the family environment that enable and sustain the dependency. Bear in mind that the psychological and behavioral impact of chemical dependency is often far greater for the family members than for the dependent person.

Crises, whether arising from outside forces or as normal developmental changes, are a normal part of family life. All crises affecting the family demand alterations or adaptation within the family system. Often people have trouble making the necessary adaptation, even in more functional families. Normal developmental issues that can create individual or family crises are events such as the birth of children, the last child entering school, the adolescence of the first child, the last child leaving home, marriage of one of the children, death of a family member, and aging. Crisis resolution in one developmental stage becomes the foundation on which the next crisis is met and becomes the basis for both individual and family growth. The more functional a family, the better these crises can be used for further growth. Less functional families remain stuck in a developmental stage because they don't have the resources to meet the presenting challenges. Characteristic of the chemically dependent family is that their interpretation of these naturally occurring developmental challenges threaten its stability, and members tend to overreact in attempting resolution.

COUNSELOR ROLES

The counselor can function in many roles in helping families. For example, it may be necessary to take immediate action to save life, to protect someone's well-being, to prevent the commission of crime, or to comply with the law in critical and urgent family situations. With the family, the counselor must observe, assess, and nonjudgmentally describe the nature of the interaction in the family system. To enable families to recognize and to better understand what is happening in their system, the counselor may also function as a teacher or an instructor.

The effective counselor creates and maintains a safe environment for change, in which people can risk being different and trying new behavior. The counselor might guide the family members toward change by helping them to gain awareness of dysfunctional behavior and explore alternative behavior, to communicate more effectively, and to determine which facets of the system the family agrees to change.

Family therapy sessions can become quite volatile. Therefore, from time to time the counselor may need to act as an umpire and insist on a time out for out-of-control sessions. Members will likely require some training and coaching in interacting and communicating their needs to each other. The family will need help in identifying the nonverbally agreed-on patterns and behaviors that usually are implied rather than explicitly stated and that frequently lie outside the awareness of family members.

The counselor may function as a facilitator in helping the family make changes. The dysfunctional rules that misuse or abuse family members within a rigid framework must be changed to rules reflecting a framework that allows self and family growth. The counselor will likely need to help the family identify and plan for new limitations, and modify rules, boundaries, and rewards for change.

It is human nature to continue a behavior as long as it provides some reward, no matter how pathological that reward may appear. Adherence to the existing system rules or behavior patterns has rewarded the individuals and the family unit. For example, maintaining rigidity avoids conflict. Unwillingness to confront unacceptable behavior avoids disapproval or rejection. Giving up individual uniqueness provides security. To recognize the necessity for changing a rule, the family and its members must see how adhering to a particular rule or set of rules has resulted in reward.

The counselor may need to help family members discover the ultimate reward of making a rule change. Every change in the family affects the equilibrium of the entire family system. Therefore, family members need to be encouraged and supported through the change. Consideration must also be given to the context within which the family's problems are presented: the time, place, and situation of a particular family interaction. Family members face different developmental tasks at different stages or times in their lives. A family may have one set of rules and patterns for behavior at home and another set for school, the workplace, or grandmother's house. The situational context is the combination of circumstances at a specific time.

PITFALLS IN FAMILY COUNSELING

Even in the best of circumstances, counselors can run into difficulty in working with people. The following list, although certainly not all inclusive, notes some of the more common pitfalls:

1. When too many data are provided by family members at once, not enough time is available for the deeper exploration necessary for effective counseling. The counselor needs to place the focus more on the process of what is occurring in the family, than on the content of the complaints.
2. A counselor's reluctance to encounter resistance can result in not meeting issues head on. Taking chances, upsetting family balance, and risking possible outbursts are often necessary to promote change.
3. A counselor eager to see quick results may attempt to push change before the parties are ready. The counselor must objectively explore whether the impetus is part of his or her own agenda rather than the family's.
4. The counselor, for whatever reason, may be unable to maintain a basic respect and caring for the family members or may tend to side with one family member against another. In that case, a referral to another counselor should be made.

5. The family may be reluctant to change. The counselor needs to keep in mind that change is scary and sometimes difficult, particularly from long-lived patterns of interaction. The family needs to move through a process of gradual assessment and change in a safe atmosphere, at their own pace, and only by their decision to change.

6. Despite indicating that they want change, the family may not engage in it. It must always be remembered that the counselor is a facilitator of people doing their own changing. If change is not happening, the counselor may express his or her concern and terminate until a later time when the family is more motivated, or refer the family elsewhere.

7. The counselor may take a magic healer or judge role. In these instances, the counselor needs to look at his or her own ego needs.

8. The counselor may become part of the dysfunctional system by getting involved in the family conflict. Again, the counselor must assess his or her own reasons for getting hooked in.

9. The counselor may not take care of him- or herself or maintain personal recreational pursuits. This can result in getting overinvolved, in allowing client contacts at other than scheduled sessions, or in taking on too many clients. The counselor needs to be fully aware of his or her own boundaries and unresolved issues, and must set limits with the clients.

10. The counselor may not accurately assess his or her professional limitations and may get involved beyond his or her level of expertise or may try to be everything to everyone. Such errors can be extremely detrimental both to the family and to the counselor.

EXERCISES

1. Name two defenses family members may present with regard to (a) the seriousness of an existing addiction and (b) their participation in the family's dysfunction.

2. In what manner might the therapist confront these defenses?

3. Describe two examples of the counselor becoming immersed in a family's dysfunction.

4. Name three ways in which a therapist's overinvolvement could be detrimental to a family, and three ways it could be detrimental to the therapist.

5. Describe two examples of how the seriousness of consequences from the chemically dependent's behavior might be unrelated to the quantity and frequency of alcohol or drugs consumed.

6. Describe three family situations in which a child's "problem" would serve to stabilize a marriage.

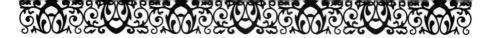

Chapter Eleven

The Family Recovery Process

The counselor must help family members recognize that treatment for chemical dependency is not a magic cure-all for the dependent, nor will it solve the family's problems. The family must realize that chemical dependency is a problem not only for the dependent, but also for the entire family. When a chemically dependent individual presents for primary treatment, the counselor should make every effort to encourage the family to enter concurrent family therapy.

There may be, on the surface, some improvement in family functioning after treatment of the chemically dependent. However, unless the other family members participate in a recovery program of their own, the critical underlying relationship problems will continue to exist and will likely be carried into another generation.

RECOVERY FOR THE CHEMICALLY DEPENDENT

Chemical dependency is, by generally accepted definition, "a disease characterized by relapse." The family must be made aware that recovery for the dependent takes time and that relapse is always possible. According to Gorski and Miller (1986), at least 20% of those who do make it have at least one relapse before achieving stable recovery. Most relapses occur within the first 90 days following treatment. Chances of a stable, long-term recovery do appear to increase with family involvement in treatment. The probability of a long-term recovery improves with each successive year of abstinence. However, some people relapse after long periods of abstinence.

Family members readily become discouraged if and when the dependent person has a relapse, or a return to use. Emphasize with family members that a relapse is not necessarily the same as failure. Many chemically dependent people suffer from what I call "terminal uniqueness." That is, through treatment they can gain enough insight into the negative consequences of their dependency on themselves and on those around them. However, somewhere from within their lingering denial system a little voice says, "I'm different. Now that I understand all this, I can control my use." Thus their venture back into active dependency can provide the dependent with the evidence needed to believe what the counselor has presented in treatment. During a period of drinking or drug use following treatment, the dependent can discover that negative effects are returning. This can be convincing evidence that he or she indeed is not so different. However, a significant number of people will never recover. Nevertheless, the family members need to begin their own recovery.

Chemical dependency has a progressive and chronic nature. That is, its onset is long, progression is gradual, and the person adapts emotionally and biologically to the disease. Stress to families that abstinence alone is *not* recovery. Abstinence only stops the disease progression. With chemical dependency, as with any chronic disease, people begin to adapt their lives to the illness. In other words, the effects of the disease shape attitudes, values, and behavior. Recovery thus involves a gradual adaptation of lives to wellness.

Gorski and Miller (1986) has outlined a fairly detailed course of recovery for the chemically dependent. They emphasize that addiction, recovery, and relapse are all progressive. At any point in time, once active addiction has ceased, one is either in a recovery process or a relapse process. Successful recovery requires following a diligent, ongoing plan of action. Therefore, when relapse does occur, it is usually not because of something the dependent personally did but rather something he or she did not do in developing and/or following a recovery strategy.

If an individual is going to be successful in recovery, once chemical use has ceased the first step must necessarily be the acceptance of the disease. Acceptance incorporates more than just admitting that chemical dependency is a problem. Acceptance is an internalization of not only a recognition of the problem but also that the individual has become comfortable in that role. According to Gorski and Miller (1986), acceptance involves three elements: (1) that chemical dependency is the problem, (2) that total abstinence is necessary for long-term recovery, and (3) that a commitment is made to an ongoing, lifelong recovery plan. If any one of these three elements is missing, relapse is likely to occur. The third element is the one most often missing after initial treatment that will lead to relapse.

Gorski and Miller (1986) has also provided a developmental model of recovery for the chemically dependent. As with any development model, the various stages or phases each require certain developmental tasks to be accomplished before one can move on to the next stage. They have identified these developmental phases and specific tasks as follows:

1. *Pretreatment* is associated with the motivational crisis that brings the individual into treatment. That motivational crisis could be based on legal requirements, the family's intervention and coercion, a physician's diagnosis of serious drug-related health

problems, or the individual having reached a point where the emotional cost has become unendurable.

2. *Stabilization* involves recognizing the problem and beginning treatment
3. *Early recovery* covers the period through completion of primary treatment, during which the motivational crisis is emotionally and cognitively processed.
4. *Middle recovery* is a period of one to two years wherein one begins to rebuild self-image and self-esteem.
5. *Late recovery* usually begins two to three years after initial treatment. During this period of time, it is necessary to identify and resolve long-term life problems. This is the time to work on issues of family of origin and identity, and to make a long-term personality change in which new ways of responding become habitual.
6. *Maintenance/remission* comes approximately five years following initial treatment. This involves full acceptance of the chronic nature of the disease and a need for lifelong recovery through continued personal growth.

Having successfully progressed through these stages, the dependant can find that his or her life has totally changed. At that point, noninvolvement with alcohol/drug use and old living patterns has become a given. Unfortunately, many people experience only partial recovery. They never become totally free of the self-defeating attitudes and habit patterns that accompany the disease. Their lives are better than when they were actively using, but they are not free to live normal, productive lives, because they are still crippled by self-imposed limits. They continue to be enslaved by their addiction even though there is abstinence. People in partial recovery always remain at a high risk of relapse.

RECOVERY FOR FAMILY MEMBERS

I reiterate, recovery can be accomplished by family members whether or not the dependent seeks treatment or ceases use. The recovery process for family members nearly parallels that of the dependent. That process also needs to begin with acceptance, the essential elements being that (1) each member's contribution to the dysfunction is the problem, (2) neither the cause nor cure for the dependency is the nonusing member's responsibility, (3) detachment from the chemically dependent is necessary for long-term recovery, and (4) a commitment to an ongoing, lifelong recovery plan is necessary. If any one of these key elements is missing, recovery is nebulous. Also with the family, the commitment of a lifelong recovery plan is the element most often missing when the members find themselves still living in dysfunctional patterns.

Family members most likely have also had their attitudes, values, and behavior shaped by the effects of chemical dependency. Having adapted their lives to the illness, recovery requires a process whereby their lives can be adapted to wellness, both of the dependent and of themselves. Families who expect only the dependent to cease use and make changes are setting themselves up for failure in achieving any higher level of functioning or emotional maturity. It can be anticipated that if the family members do not become involved in a recovery program themselves, the same maladaptive interactionary patterns will still exist. If only the chemically dependent individual attempts to change, little, if any, improvement can occur in family functioning. The result can be that the dependent will return to using or find it necessary to leave the family to preserve his or her recovery. Sometimes the spouse of the dependent, having done nothing to change destructive patterns, will discontinue the relationship even if the dependent remains abstinent, because he or she cannot adapt to the dependent's recovery and change. Not only will these maladaptive patterns continue among individuals in that family, but they will continue into succeeding generations. It is not uncommon to find an individual who has left a chemically dependent family or divorced a chemically dependent person only to become intimately involved with another. A case in point is a situation I encountered some years ago:

> A man, having acknowledged that he was unable to stop drinking and recognized that he was having a number of problems because of it, scheduled an appointment with me to enter treatment. As requested, his wife accompanied him to the appointment. It became evident that this man was alcoholic and could benefit from treatment. However, during the interview, the wife continually downplayed any symptom to which he alluded, or rationalized any of the behavior associated with his drinking. Further queries to the wife revealed that this was her third alcoholic husband. Both the first two husbands she had divorced after they had undergone treatment and had achieved some years of sobriety. I further learned that her father had died from alcoholism. At the conclusion of the interview, the husband suddenly became somewhat ambiguous in a commitment to enter treatment and indicated that he would phone the next day to schedule entry. I did receive a phone call from him the next day. However, his comment was "My wife and I have talked this over, and we've decided that treatment would be overkill." Attempts to get him to reconsider his decision were futile.

This wife was extremely threatened by another recovering husband. Never having become involved in a recovery program herself, she had not learned to make any adaptations to a functional style of living or a healthy relationship. To her, having this husband sober meant losing him and so she was prepared to sabotage any efforts on his part to get into treatment.

A DEVELOPMENTAL MODEL
OF RECOVERY FOR THE FAMILY

The family recovery process can also be delineated by developmental stages. I suggest that these stages parallel those defined by Gorski for the dependent.

Pretreatment Stage

The pretreatment segment encompasses the motivational crisis that brings the family or individual family members into treatment. That motivation may be physical or emotional abuse sustained by one or more family members. It may be a critical problem with one or more of the children. Or it may be simply that the erratic and volatile moods and behavior of the dependent can no longer be tolerated. Perhaps the dependent's legal problems have had an emotional and/or financial impact on the family. Any evidence of physical or sexual abuse of the children or unsafe conditions for the spouse must be immediately addressed. The counselor may need to make arrangements to either move the family to a safe environment or have the abusive dependent removed from the family home.

Stabilization Stage

The primary task at the stabilization stage is the family members' recognition that they did not cause the addiction, but are responsible for their own contribution to the family problems and dysfunction. This recognition begins their own participation in treatment and involvement in a self-help support group. The family members need basic education on chemical dependency and the dynamics of a chemically dependent family. Identifying incidents of enabling behavior can create a forum in which they can personally recognize their participation in the dependency. Family involvement in a 12-step programs is beneficial to recovery. Such programs offer a safe place where they can begin to associate and identify with others with similar problems, in which the family members can recognize their own enabling behaviors. Among those groups are Al-Anon for the spouse of the dependent, Codependents Anonymous, Alateen, and Children of Alcoholics.

Early Recovery Stage

In the early recovery period, the family members begin to emotionally and cognitively process their own motivational crisis or crises. They, too, must dispute the rationale that has so far sustained the family's predicament, and honestly assess personal behavior and interaction patterns. Taking responsibility for themselves and their own enabling behavior must replace blaming themselves and the dependent. Guilt and shame related to the internalized belief that they caused the addiction need to be brought out into the open and addressed. Training in basic living skills such as appropriate communication, assertiveness, and boundary delineation can be presented for the family to establish more effective interaction.

Family members may also have to relearn normal roles. For example, children may need to learn normal age-specific roles. Often children have been expected to take over adult responsibilities and functions. Sometimes not only will they have difficulty reassuming their appropriate role, but may be reluctant to give up the role they have been performing, which balanced the family system and gave them a sense of importance or belonging. Some children may need to be taught how to play and to live the life of a normal child.

Middle Recovery Stage

Within the middle recovery stage, the family begins to rebuild self-image and self-esteem and to establish a personal structured recovery plan. They must begin to modify ineffectual family rules and to clarify boundaries. As with the dependent, a pattern of growth should begin to become a habit and the benefits of recovery should become evident. This can be a very crucial and frightening period, because it involves making significant personality and pattern changes. This stage, can be extremely threatening for the chemically dependent if he or she has not begun treatment. However, it can also become the impetus for the dependent to seek treatment. If they have not already begun, the family can get specialized therapy for the children and training for parenting skills and appropriate methods for protecting the children from abuse.

Late Recovery Stage

During the late recovery stage, family members must begin to identify and resolve long-term life problems and to work on issues of family of origin and identity. Generational maladaptive patterns and boundary issues can be addressed. Long-term personality changes must be made so that the new ways of responding to the dependent and to each other become habitual. Focus needs to shift from the dependent's using or not using, to each family member developing his or her own life and seeking to improve the family. At this point, intimacy between the marital partners and the children can begin to be restored.

Maintenance/Remission Stage

This stage, of necessity, requires a full acceptance by each individual for the need for lifelong recovery through continued personal growth. Not being involved in old living patterns and not being preoccupied with the dependent's use or nonuse must be established beyond doubt. Further therapy can be pursued to heal old wounds and to enhance continued growth to increase levels of emotional maturation.

Family members, as well as the dependent, may achieve only partial recovery. They, too, may go only so far in their recovery process, because the dependent has ceased use or left the home, and the family situation may seem better. However, stopping here will not allow the family, individually or collectively, to become totally free of the self-defeating attitudes and habit patterns that limit a truly fulfilled life. Their lives may be better than when the active addiction was present. However, they probably still are not free to live healthy and productive lives because they are crippled by self-imposed limits and a preoccupation with the dependent's using or not using. They continue to be enslaved by the chemical dependency even though there may be abstinence.

EXERCISES

1. What kinds of situations can you envision that would prevent family members from committing to a lifelong recovery program?
2. What kind of lifestyle can you envision for family members who choose to not pursue a recovery program for themselves (a) once the dependent begins recovery, or (b) if the dependent continues using?

Chapter Twelve

Family Intervention

Throughout the last couple of chapters, family intervention for the chemically dependent has been mentioned. Because intervention can be such an effective impetus for inducing the chemically dependent to seek treatment, that process should be addressed more fully.

Out of their concern to not "hurt" anyone, people often tend to ignore or excuse irrational drug-affected behavior of family, friends, or coworkers. Unfortunately, this only results in the chemically dependent continuing in a state of self-delusion. Real caring for the dependent involves confronting each instance of inappropriate or irrational behavior and setting appropriate limits on use-related behavior.

Chemically dependent people generally have a fairly slanted view of reality, particularly with regard to the impact their use has on themselves and others. Therefore, the dependent needs to be provided with the kind of information to help him or her see reality as it really is. This can be accomplished in a genuine confrontation by significant others. The confrontation, or intervention, can be successful at any and all levels of severity of the dependency. However, success can most often be realized if the dependency has not progressed beyond middle or early late stage. Very late stage dependents are likely not to be as amenable to the family's concern. There also may be considerable cognitive deterioration at this stage, making it more difficult for the dependent to process information that is presented.

The dependent must be allowed to suffer any natural use-related consequences. Discontinuing any well-intended acts by family members to protect or save the dependent is essential even before beginning intervention. Family members can stop making excuses for inappropriate behavior or missed appointments of the dependent. This approach requires refusing to accommodate to the dependent's schedule, to purchase alcohol/drugs, to pay bar tabs and pick up bad checks, or any other action that tends to protect the chemically dependent. Friends and coworkers can also be solicited to help create the motivational crisis for the dependent. Friends can refrain from condoning inappropriate behavior. Instead, they can offer confrontive and supportive statements such as "I like you and consider you a good friend, but I don't like to be around you when you're drinking." Coworkers can suspend protective measures such as taking on additional work tasks and covering up for tardiness, absences, or poor performance by the dependent.

No matter how well intended, protective actions only support the denial and self-delusion of the chemically dependent. Dependent people typically do not seek treatment until their emotional pain is great enough. Protecting the dependent from pain, shame, guilt, hurt feelings, or consequences minimizes the chance for the dependent to recognize the problem that exists and his or her need for treatment. Everybody is responsible for his or her own choices and behavior. Irrational or inappropriate behavior need not and should not be accepted even of the dependent person.

Arguing with the dependent about the drinking/drug use only increases defensiveness and proves useless. Blaming anyone for the chemical dependency also serves no purpose. Chemical dependency is a disease, and no one is responsible for contracting it. Responsibility lies with an honest recognition, by both the dependent and family members, of the problem and in taking steps toward recovery. Threats are unproductive if there is no commitment to follow through on them. Intervention into the patterns of irrational thinking and behaving can be the effective tool for creating the motivational crisis that will result in the chemically dependent entering treatment.

The best candidates for a formal intervention are people who have a lot to lose, such as a family, loved one, or employment. Intervention on an emancipated adult, single child can be difficult because the parents usually don't have much leverage to use as "motivator." A formal intervention for an adolescent still attempting to discover personal boundaries and identity, and convinced of his or her invincibility, can also be difficult.

THE INTERVENTION PROCESS

Johnson (1986) speculates that even at their sickest, chemically dependent people can accept reality if basic principles of intervention are used and reality is presented in a receivable form. It is important to keep in mind that intervention into a dependent's use is a process; not an event in itself. It requires good planning and commitment to follow through.

The intervention attempt should use people who have meaning for the dependent. These are the individuals, most often consisting of family members, who can exert a real influence on the subject. Such people almost always need help in gaining sufficient emotional stabilization to carry out the task. Other interveners may be professionals such as physicians, counselors, or the clergy if they personally possess information that can be useful in providing information to present reality to the dependent. The information gathered should be factual evidence of physical complications or behavioral patterns. The most effective interveners, however, because they often can be the most influential of all, are employers or the members of management at the level next above the dependent person. It may be suitable for the family to involve the employer.

Intervention should not be attempted by people who are so emotionally distressed that they might harm themselves or the overall effort. Nor, for the most part, should intervention be attempted alone, although it can be done. A group of at least three or four is most effective because the individuals tend to support each other in getting the task accomplished successfully. As a team, they have the necessary weight to break through to reality.

The data presented to the dependent should be specific and should describe observed events that have happened or conditions that exist. Opinions and blaming should be avoided, along with all generalizations. Generalized opinions and blame raise the defenses of the dependent still higher and make the approach to reality more difficult.

The tone of the confrontation should not be judgmental. The evidence should be presented to the dependent in a manner that conveys respect and concern. The facts presented should be objective descriptions of use-related behavior to demonstrate the legitimacy of the concern. An expression of the interveners' feelings regarding observed specific behavior is appropriate. That expression might be to the effect that "I care about you, and I am really worried about what has been happening to you. These are the facts available to me, which will give you the reason I am so concerned." The evidence should be tied directly to consumption wherever possible, while relating specific incidents of concern. The more general information should only be used to support the examples of use.

I can't emphasize enough that the evidence of behavior should be presented in some detail, and very explicitly related to specific incidents. Presenting this factual information provides the dependent with a realistic view of his- or herself during a given period of time. Alcoholics/addicts have a tendency toward euphoric recall, remembering only the positive aspects of their use. In their deluded condition, they are out of touch with reality. Their greatest need, therefore, is to be confronted with reality. When presented with the facts of reality, no viable argument nor denial is possible for the dependent. It conveys the message to the dependent, "This is reality. Reality is not what you have been believing it was."

The ultimate goal of the intervention, through the presentation of this factual material, is to have the chemically dependent see and accept enough reality so that, however grudgingly, the need for help can be accepted. A most effective measure is to have a video camera to record and present the reality of situations to the dependent.

Eventually, the available choices acceptable to the interveners must be offered, along with limited preestablished consequences. The key person doing the confronting may say, "Because abstinence is a basic requirement, there are only a few alternatives before us. You must choose to enter the X inpatient facility, the Y outpatient center, or move out of the home. Which alternative do you choose?" The dependent must in some way be part of the decision making, to retain some sense of dignity.

Again, firmness here is necessary. The dependent's defenses can and very likely will regroup quickly unless it is clear the interveners truly mean what they say. In fact, at this point, the group should have predicted what the dependent will most likely offer as excuses for not accepting one of the choices being offered, and be prepared to counter them. Excuses such as "There's no one to walk the dog" or "I have to go to work," can be countered with "I'll walk the dog" or "We've already made arrangements with your boss for you to be off." When the intervention team is prepared in advance to respond to such excuses, the likelihood of treatment being accepted is greatly enhanced. It is absolutely imperative that the interveners follow through with whatever ultimatums or consequences have been presented to the dependent. The dependent has probably already faced a lot of threats that didn't materialize, so that he or she may not consider the intervention ultimatums to be serious.

GUIDELINES FOR INTERVENTION

Certain guidelines should be followed to ensure a successful intervention. Although it is not absolutely necessary, it is best for family members to work with a professional intervention specialist. The professional is in a position to remain objective and to direct and stabilize the team if the encounter becomes too emotional. Some intervention specialists are connected to a treatment facility, and some work independently of them. Making some preliminary queries of local chemical dependency treatment facilities can help the family locate a reputable intervention specialist. Johnson (1980) has provided instructions for conducting a successful intervention.

1. Initially, it must be established that chemical dependency or at least a serious problem with alcohol/drugs does indeed exist. This can be confirmed by a chemical dependency counselor trained in making that kind of determination. Although much more is needed to conduct a thorough chemical dependency assessment, family members and friends can often supply enough information to establish a need for treatment. Information such as amount and frequency of consumption, types of drugs used, irrational and bizarre behavior when under the influence, incidents of not remembering events while using, or being passed out can provide preliminary indication of chemical dependency.

2. The intervention team should consist of individuals such as family members, friends, coworkers, employer, or pastor.

3. The counselor should remain detached, supportive, and informative.

4. The person initiating the intervention contacts and makes arrangements for other persons to be involved with the process or to become part of the team.

5. Arrangements must be made in advance with one or two treatment facilities so that the dependent person can go immediately if he or she accepts help.

6. All persons on the intervention team must

    a. realize that their own attitude toward the dependent and the disease must change from blame and anger to concern and support

    b. understand that they will feel some guilt over their involvement in the intervention

    c. know that chemical dependency is a disease

    d. really believe they should be doing the intervention

Any individual not meeting these conditions should not be a part of the intervention team.

7. The counselor should initially screen prospective intervention participants. One angry person on the team, who does not care for the dependent or cannot get beyond the anger or blame, or is too emotionally unstable, can seriously impair the intervention.

8. There cannot be any idle threats. Each team member must stand firm on whatever ultimatum or consequence is being imposed. If people are unable to stand firm on the initial ultimatum, they should select a less drastic one.

9. It must be established that ultimatums to be offered will not result in harmful consequences for the team members. For example, involving the employer or requiring the dependent's departure from the home may economically devastate the family. Alternatives need to be determined before establishing any course of action.

10 As much as is possible, any and all excuses the addicted person may use must be covered. Being prepared to provide assurance that another family member has agreed to temporarily take over a specific chore removes obstacles for the dependent.

11. Before proceeding with the actual intervention, it should be determined if the subject is likely to be volatile and if there is any physical danger for any of the team members.

12. Those interveners who have lived with the dependent person must agree that they also need help.

Once the intervention team members have been established, an intervention most typically occurs in three phases: assessment and education, strategy planning and rehearsal, and actual confrontation of the dependent.

The intervention specialist can help team members realize that the chemical dependency is not just one of the problems of the dependent; it is the primary problem. An assessment should be made of the members' own understanding of chemical dependency, its progression, and how it has affected others at different stages. The specialist must impress on the team members that their helpful behavior in the past has only made it possible for the dependent to continue to use. Some basic education regarding chemical dependency may be necessary before proceeding with strategy planning.

Strategy planning and rehearsal for the actual confrontation is the next phase. The intervention specialist gives instructions on how to document situations or events and the team members' feelings regarding the dependent's behavior. Each team member determines what consequence to impose if the dependent refuses treatment. An adult child might refuse contact with a dependent parent. A good friend might inform the dependent that he or she doesn't want to continue the friendship as long as there is active use. A spouse might leave the home or insist that the dependent leave the home.

Individual team members may not all be (nor need they be) at the same emotional level, or willing or able to impose the same degree of leverage. The interventionist can help the team members determine at what level they can participate most effectively. Assistance can also be provided to members in rephrasing the "statements" they will be presenting to the dependent. Role-playing and/or practicing pre- sentation of their statements can be helpful. The interventionist should insist that all presentations be in written form, to be read at the actual confrontation. The actual event can be extremely emotional and if team members lose control, it can be disastrous. Having a prepared statement to read keeps the atmosphere more clinical and non- emotional.

Once the plan is established, the time and place of the actual confrontation can be set. If at all possible, it is best to arrange for a time that the dependent is not under the influence of a drug. Arrangements for program entry alternatives must be made prior to the actual confrontation. Such arrangements can be made by either the team leader or the intervention professional. It is a good idea to have at least two options for treatment available, so that the dependent has choices. If a period of detoxification is necessary, that must be an element to consider in the time frame. Transport to the treatment facility should also be arranged in advance so that treatment placement can occur immediately after the intervention presentation and before the dependent falls back into denial and euphoric recall. Ethically, however, the dependent should be advised at the beginning of the actual confrontation that he or she has the right to leave the intervention at any time.

With good strategy planning and preparation, the actual confrontation should go well. Keep in mind that because an intervention doesn't work at that particular time doesn't mean it isn't successful. Quite often it can take weeks or months for the presented reality to sink in or the imposed consequences to take effect. It is also not unusual for the dependent to want a period of testing the team members' seriousness with regard to their ultimatums. This, obviously, is why it is so crucial that the participants be able to follow through on their imposed consequences.

Unfortunately, there are times that the best planned and executed intervention does not ensure success. Some people are just not able to achieve recovery, even after multiple treatment attempts. An estimated 10 to 20 percent of the U.S. population is alcoholic or drug addicted. Only a very small percentage even seeks treatment, and only a minority is successful in achieving sobriety. Some people only make it after multiple treatment experiences.

I'm often asked why some alcoholics and addicts don't make it. I don't believe that any single factor prevents an individual from achieving recovery. Early in my work in the chemical dependency field, when I thought I had all the answers, I readily made assumptions such as "He just doesn't want sobriety badly enough," or "She hasn't paid enough of an emotional price," or some other cliché. However, experience has proven that these kinds of assumptions are much too simple. Most of the time a specific reason for one's failure is not readily apparent and cannot be determined. I have witnessed many people who were hurting deeply and who desperately wanted to get clean and sober. Despite repeated attempts, they never achieved any reasonable amount of sobriety. Many of them eventually died from an overdose or some alcohol- or drug-related illness or injury.

Family members, failing to coerce their dependent into treatment or their dependent fails treatment, sometimes feel the situation is hopeless. They need to be reminded that alcoholism or addiction is an insidious disease. It involves a complex intertwinement of neurological, biological, psychological, emotional, and spiritual elements. And the combination of these elements seems to vary for different individuals.

Failure of the chemically dependent, however, does not preclude that family members need to continue their suffering. I have seen family members getting help for themselves and learning to detach emotionally fom the dependent and his or her use. They have developed healthy lives, individually and sometimes collectively as a system, even with the dependent still in the home. It doesn't happen immediately with a decision to change. Nor is it an easy process. But it can happen.

EXERCISES

The class divides into groups for this exercise. In each group, select the chemically dependent, the intervention specialist, and members of an intervention team. Role play an intervention, (1) preparing statements for each team member, (2) develop an intervention strategy plan, and (3) confronting the dependent.

Conclusion

This text is not intended as a "how to" book on counseling families. It is intended to help provide an overview and a basic understanding of issues and dynamics in the chemically dependent family and to summarize what is involved in working with these families. Most of what I know about families I have learned from studying the experts—Bowen, Adler, Steinglass, Satir, and others. I have also learned from those family members with whom I've worked that rarely does a family fit neatly into a little niche. Each person and each family uniquely presents a complex battery of issues that can often seem overwhelming.

Working with families presents a tremendous challenge and requires considerable expertise beyond basic counseling skills. The counselor working with families should thoroughly understand family systems, developmental psychology, individual dynamics, normal family developmental life crises, and effective parenting. Without adequate training in these areas, no one should counsel families beyond only a preliminary level of helping them recognize chemical dependency and its related issues. Nor is it appropriate to work with young children without adequate training. The family therapist, if he or she does not thoroughly understand chemical dependency, should at least recognize its possible impact on family life and should refer to or consult with specialists in that area.

Glossary

complementarity Characteristic individual behavior that interlocks with another individual's characteristic behavior; a situation in which one person compensates for an apparent or perceived lacking in another.

detachment Remaining physically or emotionally connected to the family, but does not allow self to become involved in the dysfunction or the pain thereof.

differentiation of self Having the ability to be authentic and emotionally controlled while surrounded by the emotional intensity of the family system. It provides for individual wholeness, for being an independent and distinct entity, nonreactive and objective, while operating interdependently with the family system.

disengagement Physically or emotionally retreating from the family, discounting the family's importance and one's connection to it, but remaining emotionally tied to the dysfunction.

emotional dependency A high level of togetherness, involving a striving to act, feel, and think like others. The emotionally dependent person is reactive and subjective and responds emotionally to others out of self need. Emotional dependency prohibits being able to function as an individual whole.

emotional maturity *See* differentiation.

enmeshment The extreme sense of closeness, belonging, and togetherness among family members wherein individual autonomy is not possible.

fusion Bowen's term for the symbiotic process that involves wider relationships and that minimizes any chance of disagreement among family members.

homeostasis Basic characteristics or patterns of interaction that assure the stability or maintenance of the family system; a family's sense of equilibrium.

multigenerational transmission process The traits, characteristics, behavior patterns, and belief system that pass from one generation to another; the perpetuation of a multigenerational strain of emotional functioning.

overresponsibility One person assuming activities of and taking responsibility for another who appears unable to take responsibility for self; a situation of complementarity with an underresponsible person.

underresponsibility One person unwilling or appearing to be unable to take responsibility for self and allowing another to assume that responsibility; a situation of complementarity with an overresponsible person.

symbiosis A reciprocal emotional system between two people in which each person is controlled by the mandate of the system to ensure the other person's emotional comfort, as if each lives for and vicariously through the other.

References

Bateson, G., Jackson, D. D., Haley, J., & Weakland, J. (1956). Toward a theory of schizophrenia. *Behavioral Science, 1,* 251–264.

Bateson, G., Jackson, D. D., & Weakland, J. (1963). A note on the double-bind—1962, *Family Process, 2,* 154–161.

Bays, J. (1990). Substance abuse and child abuse. *Pediatric Clinics of North America, 37,* 881–903.

Beasley, J. D. (1987). *Wrong diagnosis, wrong treatment: The plight of the alcoholic in America.* New York: Creative Informatics.

Berne, E. (1964). *Games people play.* New York: Grove Press.

Bion, W. R. (1984). Experience in groups. *Human Relations, 1,* 314–329.

Black, C. (1979). Children of alcoholics. *Alcohol, Health and Research World,* Fall, pp. 23–27.

Black, C. (1981). *It Will Never Happen to Me.* Denver: MAC Printing.

Bowen, M. (1978). *Family Therapy in Clinical Practice.* New York: Aronson.

Bradshaw, J. (1988). *Bradshaw on: The Family.* Deerfield Beach, FL: Health Communications.

Burnam, M. A., Stein, J. A., Golding, J. M., Siegel, J. M., Sorensen, S. B., Forsythe, Z. B., & Telles, C. A. (1989). Sexual assault and mental disorders in a community population. *Journal of Consulting and Clinical Psychology, 56*(6), 843–850.

Cermak, T. L. (1986). *Diagnosing and treating co-dependence.* Minneapolis: Johnson Institute Books.

Chasnoff, I. J. (1988). Drug use in pregnancy: Parameters of risk. *Pediatric Clinics of North America, 35*(6), 1403–1412.

Colapinto, J. (1982). Structural family therapy. In A. M. Horne & M. M. Ohlsen (Eds.), *Family Counseling and Therapy,* pp. 112–137. Itasca, IL: F.E. Peacock.

Collins, J. J., & Messerschmidt, P. M. (1993). Epidemiology of alcohol-related violence. *Alcohol Health & Research World, 17*(2), 93–100.

Dreikurs, R. (1968). *Psychology in the Classroom.* New York: Harper & Row.

Dulfano, C. (1985). Family therapy of alcoholism. In S. Zimberg, J. Wallace, & S. B. Blume (Eds.), *Practical Approaches to Alcoholism Psychotherapy,* 2nd ed., pp. 313–352. New York: Plenum Press.

Dunkel, T. (1993). Dealing with demons of a new generation. *Drugs, Society, and Behavior,* 1996/1997 annual edition, Article 34, pp. 152–154, as reprinted from Insight, September 13, 1992, pp. 20–22, Washington Times Corporation.

Erskine, R. G. (1982). Transactional analysis and family therapy. In A. M. Horne & M. M. Ohlsen (Eds.), *Family Counseling and Therapy,* pp. 245–275. Itasca, IL: F. E. Peacock.

Ewing, J. A., & Fox, R. E. (1968). Family therapy of alcoholism. In J. H. Masserman (Ed.), *Current Psychiatric Therapies,* Vol. 8, pp. 86–91. New York: Grune & Stratton.

Ewing, J. A., Long, V., & Wenzil, G. G. (1961). Concurrent group psychotherapy of alcoholics and their wives. *International Journal of Group Psychotherapy, 11*, 329–338.

Fossom, M., & Mason, M. (1986). *Facing the Shame: Families in Recovery.* New York: Norton.

Gelles, R. J. (1974). *The Violent Home.* Beverly Hills: Sage.

Gorski, T. T. (1992). Diagnosing codependence. *Addiction & Recovery, 12*(7), 14–16.

Gorski, T. T., & Miller, M. (1986). *Counseling for Relapse Prevention,* Independence, MO.: Herold House-Independent Press.

Haley, J. (1976). Development of a theory: A history of a research project. In C. E. Sluzki & D. C. Ranson, (Eds.), *Double bind: The Foundation of the Communication Approach to the Family.* New York: Grune & Stratton.

Horne, A. M. (1982). Counseling families—Social learning family therapy. In A. M. Horne & M. M. Ohlsen (Eds.), *Family Counseling and Therapy,* pp. 360–388. Itaska, IL: F. E. Peacock.

Horne, A. M., & Ohlsen, M. M. (1982). *Family Counseling and Therapy.* Itasca, IL: F. E. Peacock.

Jackson, J. K. (1954). The adjustment of the family to the crisis of alcoholism. *Quarterly Journal of Studies on Alcohol, 15*, 562–586.

Johnson, V. E. (1980). *I'll Quit Tommorrow.* San Francisco: Harper & Row.

Johnson, V. E. (1986). *Intervention: How to Help Someone Who Doesn't Want Help.* Minneapolis, MN: Johnson Institute Books.

Kaufman, E. (1985). Family therapy in the treatment of alcoholism. In T. E. Bratter & G. G. Forrest (Eds.), *Alcoholism and Substance Abuse: Strategies for Clinical Intervention,* pp. 376–397. New York: Plenum.

Keith, D. V., & Whitaker, C. A. (1982). Experiential/Symbolic Family Therapy. In A. M. Horne & M. M. Ohlsen (Eds.), *Family Counseling and Therapy,* pp. 43–74. Itasca, IL: F. E. Peacock.

Kerr, M. E., & Bowen, M. (1988). *Family Evaluation.* New York: Norton.

Lewin, K. (1951). *Field Theory in Social Science.* New York: Harper.

Lowe, R. N. (1982). Adlerian/Dreikursian family counseling. In A. M. Horne & M. M. Ohlsen (Eds.), *Family Counseling and Therapy,* pp. 329–359. Itasca, IL: F. E. Peacock.

McGoldrick, M., & Gerson, R. (1985). *Genograms in Family Assessment.* New York: Norton.

McCrady, B. S. (1989). The outcome of family-involved alcoholism treatment. In M. Galanter (Ed.), *Recent Developments in Alcoholism: Vol. VII. Treatment Issues,* pp. 165–181. New York: Plenum Press.

McNeece, C. A., & DiNitto, D. M. (1994). *Chemical Dependency: A Systems Approach.* Englewood Cliffs, NJ: Prentice-Hall.

Meeks, D. E., & Kelly, C. (1970). Family therapy with the families of recovering alcoholics. *Quarterly Journal of Studies on Alcohol, 31*, pp. 399–413.

Nichols, M. (1984). *Family Therapy Concepts and Methods.* New York: Gardner Press.

Rivers, P. C. (1994). *Alcohol and Human Behavior: Theory, Research, and Practice.* Englewood Cliffs, NJ: Prentice Hall.

Roberts, A. R. (1984). *Battered Women and Their Families.* New York: Springer.

Satir, V. M. (1967). *Conjoint Family Therapy.* Palo Alto, CA: Science and Behavior Books.

Satir, V. M. (1982). The therapist and family therapy: Process model. In A. M. Horne & M. M. Ohlsen (Eds.), *Family Counseling and Therapy,* pp. 12–42. Itasca, IL: F. E. Peacock.

Sonkin, D. J., Martin, D., & Walker, L. E. (1985). *The Male Batterer: A Treatment Approach.* New York: Springer.

Steinglass, P. (1977). Family therapy in alcoholism. *The Biology of Alcoholism: Vol. 5. Treatment and Rehabilitation of the Chronic Alcoholic*, pp. 259–299. New York: Plenum.

Steinglass, P. (1987). *The Alcoholic Family.* New York: Basic Books.

Steinglass, P., Davis, S., & Berenson, O. (1975). *In-Hospital Treatment of Alcoholic Couples.* Paper presented at the American Psychiatric Association Annual Meeting, May.

Walker, C. E., Bonner, B. L., & Kaufman, K. (1988). *The Physically and Sexually Abused Child.* New York: Pergamon.

Wegscheider-Cruse, S. (1981). *Another Chance, Hope and Health for the Alcoholic Family.* Palo Alto, CA: Science and Behavior Books.

Wegscheider-Cruse, S. (1985). *Choicemaking.* Pompano Beach, FL: Health Communications.

Werner, E. (1986). Resilient offspring of alcoholics: A longitudinal study from birth to age 18. *Journal of Studies on Alcohol, 47,* 34–40.

West, M. D., & Prinz, R. J. (1987). Parental Alcoholism and Childhood Psychopathology. *Psychological Bulletin, 102,* 204–218.

Whalen, T. (1953). Wives of alcoholics: Four types observed in a family agency. *Quarterly Journal of Studies on Alcohol, 14,* 632-641.

Index

CREDITS

This page constitutes an extension of the copyright page. We have made every effort to trace the ownership of all copyrighted material and to secure permission from copyright holders. In the event of any questions arising as to the use of any material, we will be pleased to make the necessary corrections in future printings. Thanks are due to the following authors, publishers, and agents for permission to use the material indicated.

Chapter 1: 5: Six characteristics from *Family Therapy Concepts and Methods* by M. Nichols, pp. 18-20, 24-26, 71-72. Copyright © 1984 Gardner Press; **9-10:** Seven stages summarized from *Alcohol and Human Behavior* by Rivers, P. Clayton, pp. 211-227. Copyright © 1994 Prentice-Hall, Inc. Reprinted with permission. **Chapter 3: 25-26:** Excerpts on "Structural Family Therapy" from *Family Counseling and Therapy* by A.M. Horne and M.M. Ohlsen, pp. 1-4, 360-80. Copyright © 1982 F.E. Peacock Publishers Inc., Itasca, IL. Reprinted with permission; **31:** Excerpts from *Family Evaluation: An Approach Based on Bowen Theory* by M.E. Kerr and M. Bowen, pp. 27-33, 54-81, 94-96, 100-209, 134-140, 149-154. Copyright © 1988 by Michael E. Kerr and Murray Bowen. Reprinted by permission of W.W. Norton & Company, Inc. **Chapter 9: 100-103:** Figures 9.1-9.6 from *Genograms in Family Assessment* by M. McGoldrick and R. Gerson, pp. 9-14, 19-21, 29-38. Copyright © 1985 by Monica McGoldrick and Randy Gerson, Reprinted by permission of W.W. Norton & Company, Inc. **Chapter 11: 114-115:** Developmental model of recovery list from *Counseling for Relapse Prevention* by T.T. Gorski and M. Miller. Copyright © 1986 Herald House Independence Press. Reprinted with permission. **Chapter 12: 123-124:** Guidelines for Intervention list from *I'll Quit Tomorrow* by V.E. Johnson, Copyright © 1973 HarperCollins Publishers, Inc. Reprinted with permission.